Figures of Medicine

forms of living

Stefanos Geroulanos and Todd Meyers, *series editors*

Figures of Medicine

Blood, Face Transplants, Parasites

François Delaporte

Translated by Nils F. Schott

FORDHAM UNIVERSITY PRESS
NEW YORK 2013

This work was originally published in French as François Delaporte, *Figures de la médecine*, © Editions du Cerf, 2009.

Fordham University Press has no responsibility for the persistence or accuracy of URLs for external or third-party Internet websites referred to in this publication and does not guarantee that any content on such websites is, or will remain, accurate or appropriate.

Fordham University Press also publishes its books in a variety of electronic formats. Some content that appears in print may not be available in electronic books.

Library of Congress Cataloging-in-Publication Data
Delaporte, François, 1941–
   [Figures de la médecine. English.]
   Figures of medicine : blood, face transplants, parasites / François Delaporte ; translated by Nils F. Schott. — 1st ed.
      p. ; cm. — (Forms of living)
   Includes bibliographical references.
   Summary: "What does the infamous face transplant in France in 2005 share with the examination of "swollen faces" in Latin America in the 1930s? What does blood transfusion in Europe during the 17th century have in common with the discovery of mosquitoes as parasitic vectors in China at the close of the 19th century? And, last, how does the reconstruction of noses using skin flaps in Bologna in the 16th century relate to the opening of a forehead cyst in Guatemala in 1916? The six essays that form Figures of medicine present a wealth of symmetries. François Delaporte shows that each epistemological concern demands its own mode of engagement; problems reside not only in their objects but also in the historical situations in which they emerge. Focusing on efforts to resolve medical problems that are particular and nonetheless exemplary, Delaporte unpacks these separate cases to show how multiple actors—over long periods of time and across different geographies—must be taken into account to remove epistemological blockages that stand in the way of understanding. A remarkable contribution to the history of science and medicine, this book shows the value of historical epistemology from philosophical, historical, and anthropological perspectives"—Provided by publisher.
   ISBN 978-0-8232-4444-7 (cloth : alk. paper) — ISBN 978-0-8232-4445-4 (paper : alk. paper)
   I. Title. II. Series: Forms of living.
   [DNLM: 1. History of Medicine. 2. History, Modern 1601–. 3. Blood Transfusion—history. 4. Facial Transplantation—history. 5. Parasitic Diseases—history. 6. Rhinoplasty—history. WZ 55]
   610.1—dc23
                                                                          2012046400

Printed in the United States of America
15 14 13 5 4 3 2 1
First edition

CONTENTS

Christopher Lawrence

François Delaporte is well known to historians of medicine, particularly those concerned with epidemics and tropical diseases, and also to students of the history of ideas—especially those working on the mysteries of body and mind. His studies of cholera, yellow fever, vegetable life, and the passions are all translated from the French and have been absorbed into conventional Anglo-American scholarship. His work enjoys and deserves a wide readership not only for its substance but also because of his approach, which has a capacity to alarm scholars coming from traditional backgrounds much as the works of Michel Foucault did from the 1960s onwards. This is scarcely surprising: Delaporte was a student of Foucault's and has a deep appreciation of one of Foucault's own masters, George Canguilhem, on whose work he has extensively commented.

Delaporte might be flippantly described as an epistemology hunter. He tramps through the tangled undergrowth of historical and contemporary ideas of the body and mind and their disorders searching for the epistemological beasts to which that undergrowth gives shelter and support and on whose existence these creatures likewise depend. Put in a less florid fashion Delaporte seeks to discover the epistemological rules or assumptions (the *problematic* if you like) that govern beliefs and practices that although seemingly similar to our own are in fact quite alien and framed for quite different purposes.

With his flair for seeing difference where others might find continuity Delaporte impresses his readers in an extravagant and at times polemical manner. His skill (or knack even) of seeing in a phrase or sentence the gateway to an unexplored country brings to the reader the immediate strangeness of the land he wants to visit. Such skill resides in his careful reading of historical texts. There is a brilliant example in the first chapter of *Figures of Medicine.* Blood transfusion as practiced by seventeenth-century virtuosi such as Sir Christopher Wren is often placed at the beginning of a line that runs to modern surgery. But Delaporte brings us up short with a quote from the eighteenth-century French surgeon Pierre Dionis who considered transfusion a "horrible Project." Through an analysis of the meanings of blood and life in the early modern period, Delaporte shows the reader why Dionis—a hero of Enlightenment surgery and at a naïve guess an advocate of transfusion—could find it so appalling. Delaporte does a similar job on the strange disappearance of rhinoplasty and the multiple meanings of parasitic tropical diseases.

But Delaporte's method is not simply an archaeological tool; it is a political one, for he brings it to bear on current medical issues—history is *now.* His tirade against medical ethicists in the chapter on face transplants might well be enjoyed by historians but it is not written only for them. Between the surgeons who perform this operation and their critics, unsurprisingly, Delaporte finds a "rift." This is a Delaportian unbridgeable gulf like that between Dionis and Christopher Wren. "The ethicists," he writes, "believe they are in a position to prescribe the rules of good medical conduct because thanks to the collaboration of specialists with different backgrounds (philosophy, law, psychology, sociology, anthropology), they have an overall perspective on the situation." But whereas "the ethicists' concern inscribes itself on the register of moral reflection" and "subordinate[s] medical techniques to a metaphysics of life," surgeons "make these techniques serve a physics of life." Practical exigency trumps armchair ethics. For ethicists every "medical problem [is enclosed] . . . within the confines of cases already adjudicated." Social interest theorists will enjoy Delaporte's aside: "The ethicists' argumentation is a move to legitimize medical ethics as an academic specialty" although it is not necessary to accept this conclusion to admire Delaporte's method, nor indeed is it inconsistent to endorse his analysis but reject face transplants on other grounds.

Delaporte's work may come as a shock and surprise to new readers familiar with other ways of working but the apparent novelty of his method and interests can, from another perspective, be seen as approaching exactly the same sorts of problems that intellectual historians writing in English have been tackling for some fifty years. It could well be said that his work dovetails with what the best historians of ideas have been doing for a good while. Drawing on anthropology and sociology they have been seeking to expose the ways in which communities construct ideas and practices, teasing out the local nature, historical specificity and the social and intellectual uses of these things. Historians sympathetic to this approach and familiar with Delaporte's studies will recognize that, in its own way, *Figures of Medicine* does just this, and they will welcome it as an addition to a longstanding *rapprochement*.

Emmanuel Fournier

What do the beginnings of blood transfusion in Europe in the second half of the seventeenth century have in common with the discovery of mosquitoes as the vectors of parasites in China at the end of the nineteenth century? What do the reconstitution of noses by means of skin flaps in Bologna at the end of the sixteenth century share with the opening of a sebaceous forehead cyst in Guatemala in 1916? And what is there in common between the examination of a face transplant in Amiens in 2005 and the examination of a "swollen facies" in South America in the 1930s? Certainly not what, on the basis of thematic analogies between the texts of *Figures of Medicine*, one might at first be tempted to think—yet it is precisely in such a critique of analogy that we have to look for one of the keys to the book's unity.

Taking Recognition for Knowledge

These six texts present a profusion of symmetries, and they abound with examples of the kind of pollinations thanks to which the importation of a concept or a belief into an unrelated field helps to solve a problem. But when they are applied blindly and without taking into account the specificity of the area of research in question, symmetries and analogies end up causing more problems than they solve—and in each story, such secondary problems prompt what makes this book what it is. "The idea to have the known shed light on the unknown rarely bears fruit." By bringing together examples from extremely different horizons, the chapters of this book show that most often the choice of shedding light on the unknown by what is already known leads to impasse. In this epistemology, inappropriate solutions become veritable obstacles to solving problems. And beliefs, which are a kind of imperfect solution, figure prominently among these blockages to overcome. No doubt the most intractable are the beliefs vouched for by science, which is not exempt from groupthink and partisan judgments. It then takes many people—sometimes decades, working in different countries and contexts, and several transformations of a problem—to ensure that, one by one, all epistemological blockages that stand in the way of the problem's solution are removed.

The creation of a concept or its importation into a field that is not its own may certainly mark an opening, but they constitute the most important obstacle to the elucidation of a problem when we follow the concept in all its developments, some of which turn out to be inappropriate to the specific situation in which the problem under study poses itself. For François Delaporte, each epistemological problem contains its own mode of resolution, and if there is a unity to these problems, we need to look for it in this specificity and not in a common method of resolution they might harbor. This amounts to saying that the richness of problems resides in the richness of their objects but also in the richness of the reality and the situation in which they pose themselves. The problems of transfusion and of transplants pose themselves because individuals find themselves in situations beyond the reach of medical knowledge and present their particular affliction or their specific mutilation to powerless physicians who search for appropriate solutions. In the case of problems in parasitology, which owe almost everything to the tropical nature of the geographical regions in which they come up, the environment becomes the decisive factor. Problems do not randomly come up, they pose themselves in a certain location, they concern objects that exist in this environment and that can be found only there. The conditions of their existence or their appearance is linked to this or that environment. The conditions of the visibility of objects no doubt also rest on a theoretical problematization: there can be no question of lapsing into empiricism and of supposing that nature is itself constituted as a set of scientific objects. We would be wrong to imagine that all we would have to do to describe nature would be to listen to it. Yet if it is not enough to open our eyes to capture objects, it is not enough, either, to close them to correctly perceive these objects in the light of the mind. Problems are formulated and finally solved by an "armed gaze" because scholars find themselves caught up in an original experience, an experience that takes place in the very places where the objects are found and that puts them in contact with the richness of these places. Scientists are obsessed with a problem because they are there, on location. They are the thought of a place, and this place finally gives them the solutions to their problems, solutions another place could not have given.

As should be clear by now, the title of this book does not aim to turn already famous physicians into eminent figures but instead to underline, under the heading *figures*, cases of problem resolution that are particular and nonetheless exemplary. Sometimes we have to follow these cases to different places before we see them unravel. And as this itinerary establishes unexpected relations between people working in different places, the problem undergoes a transformation in each location. The transfusion technique develops in a back and forth between England and France. The history of nasal reconstruction techniques seems to begin in India but takes us back to North Italian society in the sixteenth century and to the work of Tagliacozzi. We are transported by mosquitoes from China, where Manson confronts filariasis, to Cuba, where Finlay faces yellow fever, and to India, where Ross studies malaria, to discover the conditions that were necessary for an understanding of the role mosquitoes play in parasitic infections. The history of onchocerciasis and its vector takes us with O'Neill to Africa, then with Robles to the coffee plantations that stretch along the slopes of Guatemala's volcanoes. The problem of trypanosomiasis develops with Chagas in Brazil but transforms and resolves itself with Romaña in Argentina. And Delaporte follows them everywhere; a historian in the field who seeks to open the history of medicine to epistemology, a nomadic epistemologist who seeks to find the historical solution of each situation and immerses himself in the places where his authors were first absorbed by the problems they had to resolve.

From Rationalizing to Taking One's Chances

To devote such attention to the environment of the objects under study is to presuppose a demanding gaze. While theory can lead to error when it pushes for the construction of inappropriate solutions or analogies, the "milieu" furnishes a wealth of occasions for false solutions. In this domain, the epistemology of *Figures of Medicine* won't be fooled. It takes us along in an investigation that constantly questions the truth of received wisdom, an investigation that quite often has to recognize this truth to be partial and thus to be a nontruth. "The false can take the place of the true, but it is not a moment of the true." Even more seriously, a half-truth, since it already gives satisfying explanations of a good number of phenomena, constitutes a conceptual blocking of the "true" truth that would provide the clear and full explanation of all phenomena. If we avoid anachronisms and allow for a description of the play of the true and the false as it presents itself in its own time, half-truths function as errors and must be considered as such. This is why this book takes care to denounce the retrospective illusions to which those historians fall victim who prefer to see only uncertainty or imprecision where there is error. Writing the history of an epistemological problem makes it necessary to pay close attention to the form of the analysis by means of which, in a given age, medicine deciphers a pathogenic mechanism: what it sees, what it retains, what it latches onto.

In consequence, the epistemologist's work consists in showing where there are blockings and in seeking to find out why they are there, without letting oneself be impressed by the plausibility of scientists' descriptions of what they do and the reasons they provide. These reasons and the prohibitions due to which medical science at certain moments turns away from what it will later accept are the object of Delaporte's meticulous and admirable dissections. Re-establishing the truth sometimes demands showing that chance or superstition intervene where scientists' narratives rationalize. From one text to the next, it seems that reasons are often just alibis or fictions brought forward to justify experiments, to mask ignorance, or to legitimize beliefs. Physicians evoke a fictitious history to hide gaps or to justify innovations. They cover up and justify to themselves their rewriting of history. "In the history of medicine, historical reconstructions serve as retrospective justifications." One of the book's strengths lies in operating reversals to show how efforts at presentation and justification reveal ignorance and prohibitions at the very moment they seek to mask or efface them. "Through these contradictions shine conditions of human subject research that might pass as legitimate." From this point of view, it would not be illogical to consider *Figures of Medicine* an attempt to sketch a history of the reasons physicians provide for their work.

This criticism is not just refreshing. While a fictive activity works to construct a certain representation of medical action, it at the same time reveals the place occupied by the medical imaginary in this very action as well as the value of experimentation derived from it. Above all, what is at stake is a sometimes unreasonable desire to know and to understand. To understand, one must experiment. This is an epistemological necessity. And as it so happens that reality does not always correspond to the imaginary, the adventure comprises an acceptance of defeat and fallibility. The history of medicine here leads to a philosophy of risk. "Prudence leads to a refusal of the very conditions of knowledge, conditions that sometimes are also conditions of therapeutic innovation. . . . Whether we like it or not, to attain security, it is always necessary to first take risks": the risk of transfusing blood from animals to human beings, then from one human being to another; the risk of shaping a piece of skin in the middle of the face into a nose; the risk of transferring a face from one woman to another; the risk of letting oneself be bitten by infected mosquitoes; the risk of committing errors of interpretation, etc. Experimentation no doubt is regularly justified by some hope for progress with which it is invested, and it happens (as in the case of the face transplant) that experimentation is itself a therapeutic act that is completed before it becomes an act of knowledge. But it never takes on such value unless it provokes questioning and renews problems. In this philosophy, experimentation is thus both iconoclastic and progressive, "taking sides against the law . . . only because that is the best way to make the law evolve," as Bernard Devauchelle tells us. It is clear that following this philosophy enjoins us to leave space for risk but also to leave space for improvisation. This does not mean that experimentation is an act of chance: even if it sometimes feeds on myths and phantasms, it belongs to a discipline and obeys the methods of which it is a continuation. But since in research matters no solutions are given in advance, one must improvise as musicians do.

Where Are the Limits of Living and Renewal?

An epistemology that pays attention to the richness of objects in the field and leaves space for risk and improvisation presupposes a good measure of confidence in nature and in life, even a touch of vitalism. To embark on research and experiments on the living, one must believe that noses can be repaired, even that this repair perhaps takes place all by itself, that—taking a mechanistic view—doing too much risks damaging the natural process of scarring. One must be confident that a living being will, by way of a sort of profound kinship, get used to the blood of another; that one human being will get along with the face of another; that a larva will take advantage of a vector to pass from one animal species to another. One must believe that nature can do much more than we can imagine and in a way will always surpass us in its originality. Our desire to experiment comprises the desire to see if an operation is feasible, but it is also the desire to see just how far nature can go in its as yet incommensurable liberty. There is a flavor of intrigued curiosity, of defiance even, to *Figures of Medicine*: just how far is it possible to follow and push nature?

Delaporte takes us into the field but also and above all into the middle of the profusion and tenacity of the living. Water, wine, beer, purgatives, tinctures, plant extracts are injected into the veins of animals—and it works, they go on living. Blood is transfused from a sheep to a calf, and a duck supplies the feathers for the tube used in the transfusion of blood from a calf to a human being. It is possible to make a nose from a piece of the arm, but a piece of the forehead does the job as well, and one might also take the nose from a corpse—that works, too. A larva passes through an insect to continue its life from one living being to another but it might as well have entrusted itself to a crustacean: the species has preferred the aerial to the fluvial path because at this particular time, the vermin abounds; vermin like *filaria sanguinis hominis* (the name says a lot about the agenda of some of these wormlike creatures), but others that present themselves as *pupa* or are complimented as *elegans* appear to be no less disturbing. In this world, vermin abounds but it also copies other vermin: small diptera (*Simulium Samboni, S. Dinelli, S. damnosum*) simulate black gnats. *Perstans, noctua, diurna, volvulus, medinensis, spiralis*, a scrimmage of filariae, worms and larvae of all sorts that drill through tissue and move across species and strike up alliances for reproduction, an abundance of insects that gorge on blood so they can give birth to new vermin not knowing they propagate others in the process. We are invited to a veritable verminological spectacle in which "fleas, lice, bugs, leeches, mosquitoes, and sand-flies" compete with *Glossinae* (*G. palpalis* and *G. tachinoides*) and mosquitoes (*Culex mosquito*, the hero of the story, but *Culex pipiens* and *Myzomia* as well) to forge fateful alliances with the worms. Who would have imagined that the filariae assemble in the blood as night falls, at the very time, that is, that the mosquitoes come out who might offer them a trip through the air to another living being? To understand how the disease and the future of a species link up, we must know everything about the behavior of these little beasts and about the physiology of their buccal apparatus. The history of vector theory hinges on ascertaining the number of blood meals taken by the female mosquito. And the study of medical entomology, which teems with surprises for the naturalist, becomes all the more captivating the more it articulates itself in terms of and enriches epistemological reflection.

This is the lesson of medical entomology but also of botany and medical horticulture. And in this context, it is interesting to bring together *Figures of Medicine* and François Delaporte's first book, *Nature's Second Kingdom*, in which knowledge of the animal kingdom precedes and provides a template for knowledge of the vegetal kingdom. Since grafts are first of all horticultural practices, have we not come full circle? Blood grafts, nose grafts, face grafts: the models are taken from the art of grafting plants.

> The idea is not new; and yet the account still surprises. The stump of an orange tree that feeds a vine shows that one and the same tree can take on, so to speak, different natures in its branches. It bears fruit of pleasant acidity on one stem and on another, it bears fruit of remarkable sweetness.

This is the advent of a poetic world in which strange communications between the vegetal, the animal, and the human come to the fore. A magical world in which to go against nature is still to be with nature and in nature. But also a world in which old worries reawaken. Won't the blood transfused from a calf into a man's veins communicate to him the animal's stupidity and heavy spirit? Won't the human being be transformed into a beast? And won't it be transformed into another by the face transplant or denatured into a worm by a parasitic disease? Alteration, animalization, bestialization, vegetabilization, they all seem possible as we follow these stories of phantasmatic transformations in which larvae become threads, noses potatoes, embryos parasites in the bellies of mothers: "To be precise we need to speak of the creation of a chimera or of a transfer of qualities." The imaginary that is engendered by François Delaporte's bestiary is less afraid of ontological changes than it is of chimera in which beings—half-human half-animal, half-insect half-larva, half-human half-worm—take on the characteristics of living beings from whom they have received only fragments and sow disorder among carefully made distinctions, threatening to mix everything up.

And yet it is here that analogy, purified by criticism, finds the ideal setting for deploying all its resources and denouncing without fear of confusion—at the very moment it makes them appear—the chimera of nosology, or of history and the sciences. And also for renewing further questions: in *Figures of Medicine*, a fact is not simply a fact, it is first of all the product of a framework that has made its visibility possible, and then, an entire possibility of conceptual conversion opens up with it as well. In this sense, error is of epistemological interest because it underlines the necessity of exploring these possibilities: "chance and error serve only those who know how to profit from them." Which brings us readers to the following questions: In order for the larvae of a concept to lead to the definitive solution of a problem, do they not also have to undergo a metamorphosis or let themselves be transferred to another way of confronting this problem? Do they not, in short, need the help of an other, a host or vector?

The subject matter of *Figures of Medicine* and the often technical presentation it requires confront the translator with a number of challenges. In keeping with the goal to make the work as accessible as possible to an Anglophone audience, I have opted throughout for clarity and simplicity as much as possible. Occasional notes and interpolations serve the same objective. I have drawn on existing translations of quotations whenever they were available, although these have from time to time been modified in accord with the French texts cited by Delaporte. All other translations are my own.

In translating a text that covers as wide a range of topics as *Figures of Medicine*, expert advice is indispensible, and this is the place to thank all those who have lent their support to this endeavor. I gratefully acknowledge the assistance provided by the staff at the Sheridan Libraries and Christine Ruggere at the Institute for the History of Medicine at Johns Hopkins as well as the help I received from the staff at the Library of Congress and at the New York Public Library's General Research Division and the Science, Industry and Business Library. Other, no less valuable assistance has come from Patricia Kain and many other friends and colleagues at Johns Hopkins and elsewhere. Special thanks are due to Arthur Goldhammer for his kind permission to include in this volume his translation of chapter 6 (published originally under the title "Chagas Today" in *Parasitologia* 47, pp. 319–27). Finally, I would like to thank the series editors, Todd Meyers, whose comments have been invaluable, and Stefanos Geroulanos, for their unrelenting support and Tom Lay and Helen Tartar at Fordham University Press for the smooth administration of the project.

Figures of Medicine

Animal Blood

The intravenous injection of toxic, medicinal or alimentary substances is a preliminary step toward blood transfusion. The experiments of the inventor of injection—the astronomer, anatomist, and architect of the new St. Paul's Cathedral Christopher Wren—precede those of the transfusers Lower, King, Cox, Perrault, and Denis. And the road from injection to transfusion is long and winding. At the outset, injections inscribe themselves in the context of inquisitive surgery. From there, physicians take the step towards therapeutic and dietetic injections, and they finally arrive at transfusions of blood. In the second half of the seventeenth century, medical thought oscillates between the goal of healing and savage experimentation. Most often, the former serves to justify the latter and offers a way to circumvent the prohibition weighing down on experiments on human subjects. Medical thought at the time also oscillates between the irrational and the rational. On the one hand, transfusion fully takes up a myth of regeneration; here, the therapeutic idea is rooted in a rejection of aging and death. On the other hand, an act of experimentation on animals is linked to an act of surgery on human beings. From an epistemological point of view, experiments on human beings were unavoidable. The therapeutic project—to repair a loss of blood—is of unprecedented novelty.

The Invention of a Procedure

The perfection of injection precedes and prepares the invention of transfusion. But one would be mistaken to believe that the guiding thread of this history is a therapeutic concern. From the start, one must remember that the first of the conditions of possibility of blood transfusion is the discovery of blood circulation. One must also add a series of innovations that are to be inscribed on different registers: the need for a sophisticated anatomy of the vascular system, the effort to improve the art of clysters, and the perfection of the syringe.

It has been known for a long time that blood is a vital fluid. But it is believed to be produced by the liver and to flow from the heart as from a source. Harvey discovers that the blood circulates in the body and that its movement ultimately ensures its production. This also explains the action of medication applied from the outside. Here, drugs act as if they had been absorbed through the mouth, but they act more quickly since they enter directly into the bloodstream, which distributes them to parts of the body affected by disease. Hence also the transformation of all therapeutic practices, for up to this point, physicians have restricted themselves to subtracting blood by phlebotomy; from the moment one realizes that the quantity of blood remains the same, however, the idea to add blood when there is a lack of it can emerge.

Harvey's discovery gives new impetus to the study of blood vessels, that is to say, physiology calls for a better understanding of the vascular network. In its exploration, injections find one of their first fields of application. De Graaf underlines the attraction this new technique exerts:

> With the help of this instrument, the curious will be able to discover the
> hidden roads nature maintains inside the human body and which she tries to

hide from our eyes. . . . Everyone knows the difficulties of getting to know the branching of vessels in all the different parts of the body and how much trouble professors of anatomy have in isolating all these vessels to show their principles, development, and distribution, which now, however, has become so easy to do with the help of this instrument.[1]

Introducing dyed liquids into the vessels renders the fine ramifications of arterioles visible; after its injection into the carotid arteries, the liquid traces the network of blood vessels and their connections on the surface of the brain.

A modest innovation may have helped to familiarize practitioners with injections. In a system of medicine that thinks disease in terms of disturbed equilibriums, to take care of oneself is to master an art of control. Administering clysters could answer the need to be one's own physician. It hardly needs stressing that clysters allow patients to give themselves a lavage without assistance, without effort, and without risk: "If it is thus true that lavages are the surest and most available remedy for all the great pains, am I not right to apply myself to the search for a machine with which patients could give themselves lavages without exposing themselves to any shame or any danger?"[2] De Graaf recalled the completely natural origin of this therapeutic practice: "The invention of clysters is not at all an achievement we owe to human beings but one we owe to animals who were the first to put them to use thanks to a purely natural instinct, for it is said that a certain bird that resembles the Stork, named Ibis and native to Egypt, showed humans the secret of lavages, because when this bird wants to empty its bowels, it syringes its behind with its seawater-filled beak."[3]

The clyster technique, much improved by an additional device, the piston, is an operation related to *infusions*. De Graaf rightly speaks of "infusive surgery," by which one has to understand the action of pouring medication into an organ, into the place where one hopes that it will exercise its salutary effects. Infusions are administered into the human body's various cavities: the nostrils, ears, mouth, womb, and anus. But not just these: if the patient is sick with gonorrhea, the infusion is administered into the member, since the pain must be appeased and the corrupted matter that resides in the urethra must be evacuated. Injection however—and in this it differs from

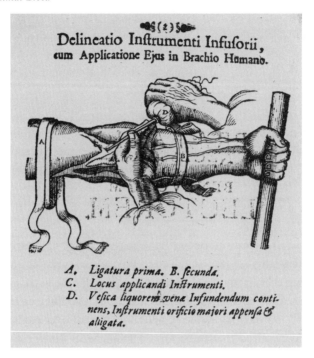

FIGURE I-I. Infusion into a vein on the arm; a bladder contains the liquid to be injected. (Johann Daniel Major, *Chirurgia infusoria*, [Kiel: Lüderwald, 1667], 2. Courtesy of Bibliothèque interuniversitaire de santé, Paris.)

infusion—involves violence. It is not a matter of letting a substance flow into an organ's orifice but of introducing it into the blood circuit—by invasion. The passage from infusion to injection is a passage from natural cavities to underlying blood vessels. The physician no longer aims at the openings on the surface of the body but at what is just underneath: the blood circuit.

In 1665 Wren publicizes his technique, which consists in making a lancet incision in the vein of the arm as for a phlebotomy and to inject the remedy with a syringe. The syringe is made up of a silver hollow needle or of a siphon, narrow at the tip and somewhat curved to better fit into the vein. At the other end there is a little bellows or a piston, which contains the medication to be injected, attached to the needle. The vein is tied in two places to make it swell. Having untied the upper ligature, the physician proceeds with the injection. The recommendation is to slowly introduce the liquid and to ease its flow with a massage that will prevent the blood from clotting.

The path that leads from injection to transfusion leads from inquisitive surgery *via* therapeutic surgery to dietetic surgery. Once injection is perfected, perfusion experiments can begin. The framework of experimentation is limited to examining the effects the injected substances have. But it

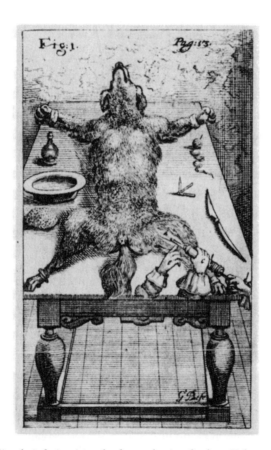

FIGURE 1-2. Simple infusion into the femoral vein of a dog. (Johann Sigismund Elsholz, *Clysmatica nova* [Coloniae Brandenburgicae (Berlin): Reicheluis, 1667], 13. Courtesy of Bibliothèque de l'Académie nationale de medicine.)

would be wrong to speak of toxicological experiments. Inquisitive surgery seeks to surprise. The administration of poisons turns operations into spectacles. The veins of animals are injected with water, wine, purgatives, plant extracts, tinctures, caustics or poisons. If it were absolutely necessary to find anything useful in these experiments, it would have to be said that these injections are a means to identify the properties of the injected substances—hence the distinction between harmful, lethal, and harmless substances. An extract of opium injected in a dog's vein plunges it in a deep sleep. A decoction of arsenic or of spirit of niter (nitric acid) provokes vomiting and the death of the animal. Injection with oil of vitriol (sulfuric acid) in turn does not suffice to kill the dog: the solution seems to augment its appetite. Fracassati distinguishes himself by injecting spirit of vitriol into a dog's vein; he provokes an epileptic crisis. Depending on the solution injected, these operations purged, intoxicated, or revitalized different creatures.

In contrast to inquisitive surgery, salutary surgery can have a therapeutic or dietetic purpose. This kind of surgery returns within the purview of Perrault's great project concerning the use of medication. The practice is guided by a concern with efficacy. Its advantages over the administration of remedies via natural pathways seem obvious. Substances that are ingested lose part of their force or are altered before they can mix with the blood. Furthermore, they undergo a profound change when they are digested. It can also happen that the state of a patient does not allow for ingesting even the smallest of remedies. Thanks to injection, the medication mixes with the blood that carries it to the organs: "The end for which surgical infusion was invented and the reason why medication is injected into the veins is to quickly mix the medication with the blood and to carry it to the heart without diminishing its force, from there to distribute it throughout the machine of the body and to quicken and reinforce its action."[4]

A therapeutic aim accounts for the transition from dogs to human beings. Ettmüller speaks of a few injections that are crowned by success. A soldier has an ulcer on his left leg; after an incision into the femoral vein, an injection of plantain solution is administered. A second patient, who has a fever, undergoes the same operation. A third, who suffers from scorbutic cachexia, is injected with a decoction of scurvy-grass. Finally, a soldier who displays ulcers and tumors is injected with several grams of scammony resin infused

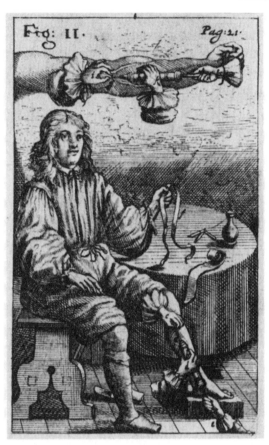

FIGURE 1-3. Simple infusion into a human subject's arm and leg. (Johann Sigismund Elsholz, *Clysmatica nova* [Coloniae Brandenburgicae (Berlin): Reicheluis, 1667], 21. Courtesy of Bibliothèque de l'Académie nationale de medicine.)

in spirit of Guaicum. Most of the time, injection is presented as a remedy of last resort, useful when the patient's digestive apparatus can neither receive medication nor produce the food necessary to strengthen the blood: "Is it not better in this extremity to attempt something so extraordinary rather than to entirely abandon this poor patient? . . . This operation applies to the most desperate afflictions."[5]

The invention of transfusion is undoubtedly in line with these techniques of injection. To be precise, we'd better say that this new operation appears as an extension of dietetic surgery. It is common to inject nutritious substances into animals' blood. Purmann, a Breslau surgeon, practices injections of broths and of warm milk. Denis injects a small quantity of milk that mixes with the blood right away. Lower shoots several alimentary extracts in the same fashion. He notes that the blood of different animals agrees with several injections of wine and beer. If these liquids could be injected without danger to the animal, the same had *a forteriori* to be true for blood, the nourishing element *par excellence*. But physicians do not overlook that discharged blood tends to coagulate as soon as it is exposed to air. Lower looks for another way of transferring blood into a patient's vein—hence the invention of transfusion. This operation allows him to avoid the obstacles tied to blood's immediate coagulation. To begin, he has to try to transfuse the blood of an animal:

> I thought it much more convenient to transfer the unimpaired blood of
> an animal, which was still alive and breathing, into another. I thought this
> would be more easily effected, inasmuch as the movement of blood through
> its vessels is so rapid and swift, that I had observed almost the whole mass of
> blood flow out in a few seconds, where an outlet offered. Taking hope from
> this, I turned mind and hands to put the matter to a practical test.[6]

The move from injection to transfusion is decisive. The technique is close to that of injection: a vein of the recipient is opened to fit into it a silver or ivory tube that points upward. The same operation is carried out on the donor, but the tube points toward the lower part of the vein. Finally, the tubes are joined by inserting one into the other. It seems Lower is the first to transmit blood from jugular to jugular by means of tubes that are well fitted to the veins of two dogs. But blood coagulation still blocks the operation: "Seeing the blood clot at once in the tube and block its own passage on account of the slow movement of the venous blood, I soon began to try another way, and guided, as it were, by nature herself, I finally determined to transfer blood from an artery of one animal into a vein of a second; and by this new device to extend the circulation of the blood beyond the boundaries prescribed for it [by nature]."[7] Since transfusion is concerned with replacing the same quantity of blood as that which has been drawn, phlebotomy is transfusion's complementary operation.

As of February 1666 Lower has opened the way for transfusions. The following year, the experimental protocol is imported into France. Denis is assisted by the surgeon Emmeretz and Perrault by the surgeon Gayant;

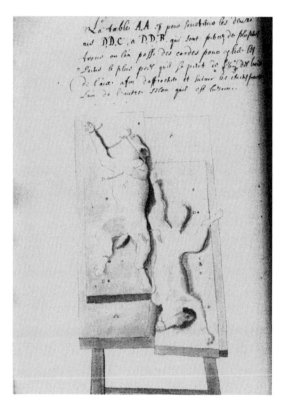

FIGURE 1-4. The dogs are tied onto planks that rest on a table. To operate the transfusion from the femoral artery of the donor to the femoral vein of the recipient, the siphons are fitted into one another. This drawing was to illustrate Claude Perrault's *Essais de physique ou recueil de plusieurs traits touchant les choses naturelles* (Paris: Coignard, 1688), 4: 406–8; it is to be found in the minutes of the *Académie des sciences. (Procès verbaux–Registre de physique*, vol. 1 [Paris: Académie des sciences, 1667 and 1668], folio 216. Courtesy of Académie des sciences, Institut de France.)

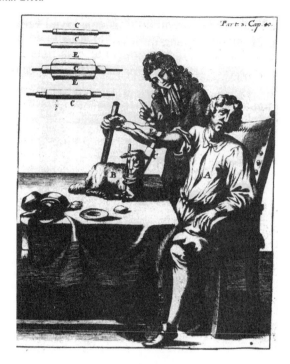

FIGURE 1-5. A physician transfuses the blood of a lamb into a patient. (Matthias Gottfried Purmann, *Lorbeer-Krantz oder Wund-Artzney* [Frankfurt and Leipzig: Rohrlachs, 1692]. Courtesy of Bibliothèque interuniversitaire de santé, Paris.)

both need assistants who are well familiar with phlebotomy. Phlebotomy's procedure, after all, coincides with the surgical acts that define transfusion, the opening of the veins of donor and recipient. Perrault's first experiment takes place on January 22, 1667, at the Academy of Sciences, which then had its seat at the king's library. The operation consists in transfusing blood from the femoral artery of one dog into another dog's femoral vein. The quantity of blood transfused is in doubt because the siphons are badly constructed. Some days later, Perrault proceeds to a transfusion from one dog's carotid to the jugular of another: the recipient dies, and its right ventricle and superior *vena cava* are found to be filled with clotted blood. Denis begins his experiments some months later.

Physicians transfuse the blood of different animal species: sheep, calves, dogs are made to contribute. King, for example, pairs a lamb with a calf or a dog. Perrault and Denis proceed to modify the procedure as it has been practiced in England. They transfuse from vein to vein but they also use the donor's carotid or femoral artery. Denis pairs animals of the same species to make the blood flow from one animal's femoral artery to the jugular vein of the other while a third tube poured onto a plate about as much blood as it received from it.

Blood clotting in the tubes or in the veins of the recipient animal is a frequent cause of setbacks. To avoid the inconveniences caused by the rigidity of metal tubes, practitioners substitute more flexible tubes, the carotid artery of a cow, say, or its ureter. De Graaf chooses a tube made of duck feathers that are joined together: "This machine is much more appropriate for making a transfusion of blood from one animal into another than is the silver or copper instrument used in Paris for this procedure, for with this instrument, whose middle part is flexible, the animals are not obliged to keep their bodies in the same position as they are with the Paris instrument, whose middle part is rigid and does not bend at all."[8]

Boyle has recommended precision. Accordingly, Perrault suggests that the test animals be weighed to make sure of the quantities of blood given and received. One dog is placed on each of the two sides of a balance; the dogs are attached to planks and each is fitted with a siphon, which is ready to be joined to the other dog's siphon. The addition of weights brings the balance into equilibrium. After the transfusion, a new weighing is undertaken to find out how much blood an animal has received. Perrault recommends attention be paid to the variations of the recipient's pulse, to emissions of urine or of excrement. It is also necessary to have several replacement dogs ready in case just one dog should prove insufficient.

From Animals to Human Beings

Very quickly, the French adapt the technique they have taken over from the English and tested on animals for use on humans. There is, however, no doubt that no human being could be sacrificed to save another, never mind sacrificed for the purpose of experimentation. Denis quickly outlines the principles that guide his therapeutic practices. The therapeutic goal determines the choice of donor animal. Put very schematically, the different qualities of the vital fluid account for its powers. By dampening the heat and fermentation of blood that is too hot, cold blood slows down the latter's impetuosity and the production of animal spirits; it offers the therapeutic virtues of a sedative. Inversely, by overexciting blood that is heavy, stagnant, and as if stiff with cold, warm blood speeds up the latter's movement and the production of spirits; it offers the therapeutic virtues of a tonic. In this sense, blood transfusions can constitute a set of medical responses appropriate to different pathologies. Once this conception is taken to its logical conclusion, nothing stands in the way of endowing animal blood with the qualities hoped for. All that needs to be done is to impose on the animal a dietary regimen such that it results in offering the quintessence of this or that therapeutic virtue.

On June 25, 1667, Denis undertakes the first transfusions on a fifteen-year-old boy. The boy displays memory problems, is in a state of great fatigue, and has a fever. For the physician, these symptoms have to be attributed to the presence of black and viscous blood. In addition, the preceding treatments have contributed to a deterioration of his situation. He has had his blood let more than twenty times. Stagnating in the vessels, his blood has lost its movement and its heat—hence the young patient's apathy, due to a lack of animal spirits. He quickly has to have a transfusion of a fluid to repair this damage—the blood of a lamb, which is to act as a ferment. The operation is to facilitate the return of life thanks to a production of animal spirits. The boy regains use of his limbs, his appetite returns, and his health improves:

> I ask't him now and then, how he found himself, he told me that during the operation he had felt a very great heat along his Arm, and since perceiv'd himself much eased of a pain in his side, which he had gotten the evening before by falling down a pair of staires of ten steps. He was also in little time perfectly cured of his somnolence and about ten of the clock he was minded to rise and being I observed him cheerful enough I did not oppose it and for the rest of the day he spent it with much more liveliness than ordinary; eat his Meals very well without falling asleep and shewed a clear and smiling countenance.[9]

The account of this first success is met with skepticism. The beneficial effects that follow the transfusion could be attributed to a different cause, in this particular instance a salutary shock tied to the fear of such an operation: "When we gave him the blood of this lamb, the vivid apprehension he had of a remedy that is uncommon and whose outcome could not but appear very doubtful to him bestirred his spirits and relieved them of the difficulties that had prevented their distribution; from this relief then followed all the advantages that are attributed to transfusion."[10] Denis points out that his patient had been unaware of the nature of the treatment he was to undergo and therefore had had no occasion to be in the least apprehensive. The fright argument is nonetheless not without importance: Denis makes it himself, albeit for a diametrically opposed reason. He jettisons the idea of experimenting on inmates who were condemned to death because the fear they would feel could lead to the failure of the procedure—and yet his detractors would quickly put down this failure to the transfusion alone.

Experimenters base their practice on two medical doctrines. The first is iatromechanism, namely to the extent that transfusion as a therapeutic gesture consists in reestablishing the equilibrium of fluids. For Lower, the principal advantage of the operation lies in the reparation of a loss: "If blood is withdrawn or is lost from bodies in good condition, by unsuitable venesection, trauma, or haemorrhage of any kind, in such amount as to require immediate replenishment from elsewhere, I have no doubt that the blood of animals can safely and advantageously be substituted in the place of that which has been lost."[11] For Denis, well-tempered blood is a sign of health. Transfusion is to allow for the restoration of the blood's normal temperature: "If a hot Blood can reinfuse new strength into that which languisheth with coldness, such blood as hath colder qualities, may also check the Ebullitions and Tumults of that which is overmuch chafed."[12] The second doctrine is iatrochemistry because spoilt blood could easily be changed by the animal blood's qualities:

> For as the roughest Wine may be sweetned, the fowlest clarified, the weakest become stronger, the Oylie rid it self of its fatness; in a word, that which is decay'd may be amended by mixture of certain liquors known to those that have the secrets of them, and practise the same every day; in like manner, 'tis reasonable to conceive that blood too thick may be refined and subtilised, that

too subtle be fixed and incrassated, that too hot be temper'd, that too cold be heated, and all this by the mixture of other sorts of blood, the particular qualities whereof are known to the Physitian who prescribes the *Transfusion*.[13]

Just as meat from animals of different species does not all taste the same, so their blood offers particular virtues. The distinct properties of animal matter have to be kept in mind, provided that these differences apply only on the dietetic register. The question of blood's nutritional value has nothing to do with the play of sympathies or antipathies between different sorts of blood. Transfusers neither believe in affinities between bloods of animals of the same species, nor do they believe in the incompatibility of the bloods of animals of different species. The vital fluid is beneficial insofar—and only insofar—as it is food. Blood thus has to be aligned with the products human beings derive from the animal world to feed themselves. Not completely so, however, for blood is seen as a food so subtle it does not need to be digested, as flesh does, before it is assimilated. Put differently, the donor's blood can be mixed with the recipient's directly and without the least preparation.

It might of course happen that the transfused blood deteriorates and spoils in the recipient's blood vessels. This inconvenience is of the same order as that which comes about when food enters a digestive apparatus off balance. Most of the time, however, transfusion offers nothing but advantages. It returns an exhausted body to strength. It supplements the digestive functions of a weakened organism. Transfusion imposes itself as a therapy both symmetrical to and the inverse of phlebotomy. The convention is to withdraw bad blood; instead, the convention has to become to inject good blood. Meanwhile practitioners of phlebotomy have a favorable view of the new technique. If bad blood is to be replenished, it has to be withdrawn. Phlebotomy becomes transfusion's complement.

Yet transfusions of animal blood to human recipients triggers lively criticism. From a medical point of view, these operations seem useless, even dangerous. For Lamy, all diseases with an internal cause follow from either the heat of the blood or from its impurity. Against the diseases that depend on the blood's overheating, transfusions are useless: the blood transfused is warmer than that of the patient. Against diseases that derive from the blood's corruption, transfusions are useless: the foreign blood is immediately altered by the recipient's blood vessels. On this point, Lower agrees with those of his opponents who do not believe in the operation's utility:

> Patients, whose blood is definitely putrid and has been long corrupt, or is very deeply tainted by a poisonous ferment from without, those, too, whose viscera are polluted and spoilt, as sometimes happens in cases of scurvy, venereal disease, leprosy, poisoning, or long-continued illness, cannot hope for any benefit or help from transfusion.
>
> The impure blood, in its repeated passage through the viscera, imparts to them its defects and its pollutions.[14]

Reasons for the rejection are also of a physiological order. Fear of transfusion is due to a perception of blood as the highly elaborate product of a physiological function. For Perrault, sanguification is the result of nutrition, which must follow the paths of nature. Digestion ensures the transformation of food into chyle. A final operation takes place by means of circulation. Only after thus having been altered, matured, and perfected is the blood of an animal ready to nourish it. Yet the blood drawn from an animal's veins has the same status as any other food: it must be absorbed, digested and prepared before being assimilated. The donor's blood cannot be mixed directly, without preparation, with the recipient's blood: "Alien blood will never become an animal's own and natural blood if it is not been converted into chyle in its stomach and then yet further altered, cooked and perfected in the organs to which nature has given the virtue of impregnating chyle with the true character of blood."[15]

There is a third reason to oppose the transfusion operation. It comes from medical philosophy. For the advocates of naturism, clotting in the recipient's veins is inevitable because the recipient's vein differs from the donor's like a receptacle differs from the blood's natural place. For Perrault, coagulation of the blood in the vein into which it has been received indicates the disharmony that ensues from the encounter of the matter received with the body part that receives it; the latter is only the vase that contains the transfused blood and not its natural place.

Transfusers and antitransfusers also oppose each other on a fundamental question. At first sight, the operation of grafting offers a tempting model. It can happen that a foreign branch adapts to the sap of the tree into which it is inserted. The trunk of an orange tree can feed a jasmine branch. Why would one animal's blood not be able to adapt to that of another? Blood transfusions would then work like grafts: the nourishing fluids could mix without difficulty.

For Perrault, the comparison of blood transfusion to the grafting of trees is inadmissible. Both plants and animals feed themselves, grow, and keep themselves alive, but they do not execute these functions the same way:

> It is a constant that nature does not at all expend the same care and exactness on plants as she employs on behalf of animals in whose actions she always follows the same order; what is not needed in less perfect food (like that which suffices for plants, in which we see the root serving them as mouth and stomach and even as heart) is by no means a part whose structure and temperament would have to have something so exquisite, so particular that its action could not be supplied by another part.[16]

Plants' food is drawn from the soil. A common, raw, thick nourishing sap is sufficient to feed them. Under these conditions, it is easy to understand that a vegetal graft could adapt to a foreign sap. The tree sap's rudimentary nature facilitates its rapid modification for an assimilation by the graft. This amounts to saying that the grafting procedure appears as elementary nutrition: the trunk's sap is to the branch that receives the sap what the food drawn from the roots is to the plant. In animals, however, the chyle receives the mark that the digestive apparatus leaves on it. The heart then imprints on the chyle that character of the blood that is appropriate to the animal it is to nourish. Blood has the status of a specific product, elaborated and assimilated exclusively by the organism that produces it: "Thus the parts of each animal can be nourished only by blood that was prepared for these parts; and the flesh of a dog cannot be repaired and nourished by the blood of a fox, nor can the flesh of one dog [be repaired and nourished] by the blood of another dog."[17] Perrault refuses to align blood transfusion with plant grafts because blood, unlike sap, is an *irreplaceable* fluid.

Advocates of transfusion equally refuse to align the superior with the inferior, but for an opposite reason. As far as nutrition is concerned, everything about plants appears to be simpler. Yet a closer look shows that the process of grafting is much more complex than the operation of transfusion. The sap coming from the trunk must be changed as it passes into the alien branch. This means that the plant graft is a mechanism of sap elaboration analogous to the mechanism of blood elaboration. Just as chyle must be transformed into blood to form flesh and bones, so sap must be modified such that its particles form mucilage that is able to feed branches from a vine or a jasmine bush. Denis refuses to align blood transfusion with plant grafts because he thinks that blood, unlike sap, is an *interchangeable* fluid.

Indeed, blood transfusion consists in the transport of the fluid from donor to receiver. This explains the status blood has for the transfusers: a liquid already elaborated, a standard product that is easily substituted. That is why blood transfusion cannot be compared to plant grafts:

> This way of changing the blood of animals seems different from grafting: for grafts convert in their nature the juice of the trunk on which they are put. . . . [I]n this transfusion of blood it seems instead that no such filtration of the animals' blood takes place. . . . It seems that the most considerable utility one could derive from this experiment is that one animal can live with the blood of another and, in consequence, that one can substitute in sufficient quantity the blood of other animals in animals that have hardly any blood left or whose blood is corrupted.[18]

There is another divergence of perspectives, in line with the preceding. For Denis, the fetus's nutrition presents a model of natural transfusion to justify the operation. This amounts to saying that nature teaches blood transfusion. If art counterfeits nature, then the operation is at the same time legitimate and without danger:

> The Transfusion of the blood of one Animal into another is sufficiently taught us by Nature it self, and it must be granted that if we ever practise the same, we shall do no more but imitate her; since whil'st she cannot yet administer nourishment to the Fœtus by the mouth, and his stomack is not fit for digestion, she makes a continual Transfusion of the Maternal blood into the Umbilical Vein of the Infant, therewith to nourish, vivifie, and encrease all the parts of the same. To have a transfusion done is nothing but to feed oneself by a path shorter than the ordinary one, that is to say, to put into one's veins blood that is all ready-made instead of taking in food that does not turn into blood until after several changes.[19]

This idea could only be rejected by Perrault. He considered blood to be an organic element indissociable from the organism that produces it for its own conservation. The mother's blood is thus a foreign blood the fetus must prepare, correct, and refine: "We can say that it is for this reason that Nature has taken so many precautions in the structure of the umbilical vessels and of those of the afterbirth, destined for the preparation of the food of animals while they are in their mother's womb."[20]

The Operation's Risks

Lower has no doubt that the invention of blood transfusion will become famous thanks to the advantages it will bring to the human species, provided it is handled prudently and skillfully. In fact, however, it becomes famous for a completely different reason. In France, transfusion finds itself very quickly associated with the death of a patient. The research subject is no ordinary patient. He displays signs of madness—at first sight a subject who offers nothing but advantages. It suffices to announce a new therapy to justify experimentation on a sick individual. But events take a different turn. Christiaan Huygens echoes the public rumors: "It would be important to make people see that diseases can be healed by this procedure, as some have wanted to attempt here [in Paris] by practicing it on a madman who, however, or so one hears, died in the end at the hands of these transfusers."[21] But let's not get ahead of ourselves.

After Denis's trials with a young man and a porter of sedan chairs, experiments begin in England. In November 1667, King and Lower transfuse a few ounces of blood from a young animal's carotid artery into a vein in the arm of their subject, a simple-minded man named Arthur Cogan, who has agreed to submit to the experiment for a few shillings.

> For there is no reason to think that the blood of other animals mixes less well with human blood than with animal blood. This view is abundantly confirmed by recent experiments of French workers, and I also found it so not very long ago in the case of a certain *A.C.*, who was the subject of a harmless form of insanity. I superintended the introduction into his arm at various times of some ounces of sheep's blood at a meeting of the *Royal Society*, and that without any inconvenience to him.[22]

The following month, in France, it is the turn of a thirty-four-year-old patient, who had for a long time already displayed unequivocal signs of madness. Mauroy runs around the Marais quarter of Paris in the nude. His disease moves the Monsieur de Montmor to compassion; he decides to come to aid of the poor man, abandoned by all, by asking Denis to administer some blood transfusions. The first operation takes place on December 19, 1667. The therapeutic idea is simple: thanks to its gentleness, the blood from a calf's femoral artery could temper the ardor of the poor madman's blood. After the first session, the man appears to be more peaceful and more moderate in his utterances. After the second session, the effects are surprising. The patient still displays a few symptoms: irregular pulse, abundant sweating, and repeated vomiting. But very quickly, the recovery is complete: he gives not a single sign of madness, makes up with his wife and goes to confession. The third session triggers the scandal. At the end of January, he falls ill. Following this relapse, his wife calls Denis. The moment blood is drawn from a vein in his foot, tremors seize the patient. He dies shortly afterward.

The events that follow are rather confusing. For some, the whole affair is a dark plot instigated by some members of the faculty of medicine who allegedly have bribed the wife to bring charges against Denis. Denis, for his part, suspects her of having poisoned her husband by mixing arsenic into his soup and then having turned on Denis, threatening to accuse him of her husband's death if he does not give her some pieces of silver. This is certainly what prompts Denis to bring the affair before the courts and to demand, in vain, an autopsy of the deceased's corpse.

Denis copies the judgment of the Châtelet court, dated April 7, 1668, in a letter he addresses to his friends in London. The judgment in the Mauroy affair does not prohibit the procedure. It strongly recommends that in the future transfusions take place under the control of the faculty of medicine. But here the text: "Whereupon it was decreed, that the widow of du Mauroy [*sic*] should on a set day appear personally, and undergo the examination upon the alleged informations; and that more ample informations should be made of the contents in the complaint of Mr. Denis: And then, that for the future no transfusion should be made upon any human body but by the approbation of the physicians of the Parisian faculty."[23] It is easy to see that in this affair Denis is the accuser and that no prohibition weighs on transfusion. But the significance of this new procedure largely exceeds the legal framework within which it was supposed to be confined.

A medical concern seems to animate the French and English projects. They present the subjects of their experiments as sick men stricken with madness, as patients that have to be treated with transfusions. This does not, however, prevent them from underlining the uselessness of the procedure in cases where the mind is affected. Lower insists on this point: "Further, in arthritic patients and lunatics, whose bodies are strong and viscera firm, the composition of whose brains is not yet spoilt, and whose blood is affected by no putrid disease, perhaps as much benefit is to be expected from the infusion of fresh blood as from withdrawal of the old."[24]

A concern with transparency appears to animate the transfusers' project as well. To elicit the consent of their research subjects by means of remuneration is to intimate that they can be held responsible for their acts. But at the same time, the physicians insist that these volunteers have lost their mind. In England, such is the case for Cogan who accepts to receive a transfusion for a little money even though he is not in full possession of his faculties. In France, such is the case for the second of Denis's transfusion subjects, a healthy man in his prime, whose behavior is truly surprising. Denis transfuses ten ounces of blood from the femoral artery of a lamb. After the operation the porter does not only refuse to take some rest, but he immediately cuts the lamb's throat, blows hard to separate its skin from the flesh, skins the lamb, and runs off to the cabaret to drink away the money he has received.

On the one hand, physicians treat madmen but declare that madness cannot be treated by transfusion. On the other, transfusions are practiced on subjects who are responsible for their acts but are shown to display signs of derangement. These contradictions reveal a desire and a fear. The desire is to experiment on human beings to see if the procedure can be performed successfully. Denis stresses that the transfusion on the sedan chair porter is undertaken "more out of curiosity than out of necessity, for the one on whom it was practiced did not show any considerable indisposition. He was a strong and robust porter of about forty-five years who for a rather modest sum offered himself to endure this procedure."[25] The fear is the fear of being seen as a physician who violates the prohibition of experimentation on human beings—hence the medical justification and the allusion to the subject's consent. Through these contradictions, it seems, shine conditions of human subject research that might pass as legitimate. On the one hand, experiments on human beings should not pose more of a problem than experiments on animals. Does not madness touch on animality? One should recall that at the beginning, the members of the Royal Society plan an experiment on a madman. They send a delegation to Bethlem hospital. But the director, Dr. Allen, refuses to furnish them with a patient for such an operation. On the other hand, the assent given by the research subject seems to set aside any idea of transgression. The acceptance of a cash compensation would count as consent to the experiment on the part of the research subject.

Denis and Lower want to know if the transfusion of blood from animal to human being can be made to work. But this experimental aim inscribes itself within the framework of mythical thought. An entire fund of old beliefs returns to the surface: the virtues of blood, even rejuvenation cures. Denis believes in the immense powers of such a practice. On this point, he is closer to Boyle than to Lower. It is well known that Boyle's enthusiasm knows no bounds: "It is intended that these trials shall be prosecuted to the utmost variety the subject will bear: As by exchanging the blood of old and young, sick and healthy, hot and cold, fierce and fearful, lame and wild animals, &c. and that not only of the same but also of different kinds."[26]

It is not surprising to see some physicians reactivate Paracelsus's theme of morbid transplantation to explore the inverse path, beneficial transplantation. It would be possible to heal not by giving away one's evil but by receiving health. The force of this phantasm is still perceptible in the eighteenth century in the *Encyclopédie*'s article "Transplantation": "We see an effect analogous to transplantation in what, according to some authors, happens to the elderly. When they sleep with young people they maintain good health for longer, stay fresh and active, and the young people feel the inconveniences of old age much sooner; this fact yet merits careful examination."[27] In the seventeenth century, a few transfusers certainly believe in the rejuvenation cure. All that is needed is to transplant the rejuvenator *par excellence*: blood, this vital fluid of so many qualities. To communicate the ardency of youth, it will suffice to infuse new blood.

Transfusion, to be sure, is an overdetermined procedure. Blood is an element without apparent form and quality. But this liquid is all the more precious as it contains all forms and qualities potentially. Organs and temperaments have their origin in blood. Denis places all positive values of nature in the blood of animals. From this point of view, human blood appears as a denatured element. If all vices flow in the veins of human beings, it will suffice to have the blood of animals flow there instead. Humans will find once more the calm, happiness, and innocence of the earliest days: "Sadness, Envy, Anger, Melancholy, Disquiet, and generally all the Passions, are as so many causes which trouble the life of man, and Corrupt the whole substance of the blood: Whereas the life of Brutes is much more regular, and less subject to all those miseries, which we ought to consider as sad consequences of the prevarication of our first Parents."[28]

Antitransfusers certainly are very much afraid of the dangers of mixing different kinds of blood. To understand the nature of their resistance, we have to return to the model of the plant graft. By finding the means to bring about new fruit, the gardener has invented the art of embellishing gardens. The idea is not new; and yet the account still surprises. The stump of an orange tree that feeds a vine shows that one and the same tree can take on, so to speak, different natures in its branches. It bears fruit of pleasant acidity on one stem and on another, it bears fruit of remarkable sweetness: "These plants, committing adultery in their own way by means of a pleasant mixing of their sap, introduce bastards along with their legitimate and natural fruit."[29]

Yet what here is little more than a pleasant analogy with gardening can easily become a matter of human justice. Zoophilia is seen as a guilty practice; coupling with animals is the worst of sex crimes. Sentences show that the animal is punished, not as guilty, but as partner in a morally reprehensible act. Killing the animal is less a symbolic punishment than it is the expression of a wish to erase from memory everything that recalls the depravation. Everything that has directly or indirectly to do with the abominable act must disappear. To cite but two examples:

> Jean le Goigneux, charged with and found guilty of having had carnal copulation with a she-ass, sentenced by decree of the Paris Parliament of December 22, 1575, to be hung, the she-ass to be knocked down beforehand in the presence of the accused; their bodies to be burnt and reduced to ashes, the accused sentenced to pay for the she-ass the person to whom she had belonged, and the trial proceedings burnt at the execution. . . . Another decree

of the Paris Parliament of December 22, 1601, that has sentenced a woman, found guilty of abominable lechery with a dog, to be hung and the dog to be attached to the same gallows; their bodies and the trial proceedings thrown into the fire.[30]

In the imagination, the mixing of bloods is identified with the crime of bestiality. For Guillaume Lamy, doctor and regent of the Paris medical faculty, transfusion is a barbaric operation. Not only does the surgeon step on the rights Providence has reserved for itself, he also attacks the dignity of the human being. Pushing the fantasy of a mixing of species as far as possible, Lamy feared new combinations. The operation of transfusion is nothing less than an act of bestialization, a sin of confusion. Underneath the rejection of blood transfusion, we have to see the fear of the human being's transformation into an animal. To be precise, we need to speak of the creation of a chimera or of a transfer of qualities. Animals have parts like feathers, wool and horns: "In their blood there must thus necessarily be particles that can form these body parts and that we do not encounter in the blood of man; and in consequence, if other little bodies in animal blood might serve to nourish man, these would always be harmful to him and would degrade, or at the least they would produce in us similar body parts." Since temperament equally depends on blood, it is to be feared that "a calf's blood being transfused into the veins of a man would also communicate to him the animal's stupidity and brutal inclinations. . . . A man who would have received an animal's blood in his veins would become heavy and oppressive of spirit and would cast off his own inclinations to take on this animal's."[31]

Clearly the choice of individuals who show signs of madness reveals not a therapeutic goal but an intention that is properly experimental. All that is needed to obscure the goal of blood transfusion, to establish it as practicable in human beings, is to present the operation as a cure. Not entirely, though; some decades later, Dionis loses sight of the transfusers' true goal. He returns to the properly medical argument and inverses the order of factors: transfusion does not cure madness but provokes it. There's more: Dionis rejects transfusion because it picks up on the art of prolonging or rejuvenating life and on the fable of Pythagoras. At the same time, the Châtelet judgment that has placed the operation under the control of the medical faculty fades into the background and gives way to an apocryphal judgment of the Paris Parliament according to which blood transfusions are prohibited under pain of corporal punishment. The eighteenth century subscribed to the judgment of the man who had been chosen by Louis XIV to teach, in the King's Garden, anatomy according to the circulation of the blood. Dionis concludes his *Course of Chirurgical Operations* with this judgment without further appeal:

> They perform'd several of these sorts of Operations, which, according to them, were to have been attended with an extraordinary Success; but the fatal End of these miserable Victims to Novelty, in one day destroy'd the mighty Opinion which they had entertain'd of their Notion; for their Patients became senseless, distracted, and afterwards dy'd. . . . Never was any Arrest more seasonably published than this, to destroy the Prepossession of these Innovators, and prevent the course of this Operation, which would have prov'd of pernicious Consequence, with regard to brotherly Love and Religion, if they had been suffer'd to perform it from Man to Man, which was the end they proposed. But those who invented this horrible Project are dead, and 'tis it self almost buried in Oblivion, and though I mention it now, 'tis only in order to rank it amongst those Operations which ought never to be practis'd.[32]

Fabricating Noses

The history of rhinoplasty calls up the history of vaccination. Just as the English import the practice of inoculation from Turkey at the beginning of the eighteenth century, so they bring back the practice of repairing noses with a forehead skin flap from India at the end of that century. But the developments or extensions are different. Jenner first perfects inoculation and then substitutes vaccination for inoculation. Yet the Indian method of nasal reconstruction leads to a reactivation of a variant of the autotransplant, namely the arm flap technique perfected by Tagliacozzi at the end of the sixteenth century. Taking their cue from the imported Indian method, European surgeons rediscover the Italian method. Speaking very schematically, it would not be wrong to say that these two procedures are equivalent as to both the surgical mode and the results. Yet the essential question is why European academics neglect rhinoplasty throughout the seventeenth and eighteenth centuries. What has happened for the arm flap technique to be obscured for such a long time? The versions contemporaries give of the history of its rediscovery are not convincing. New threads must be and are found, but they are so disparate that it is necessary to tie them together into a fabric of empirical knowledge that ends up in a system of thought indifferent to the unheard-of novelty of Tagliacozzi's art.

Chronology of Events

In the ninth chapter of book VII of his treatise *Of Medicine*, "The operations necessary in a want of substance in the ears, lips, and nose," Celsus writes:

> Defects in these three parts, or in any other that may be equally small, admit of cure: in parts of greater magnitude the cure is either altogether impracticable, or leads to so much deformity, that of the two the previous state was the least unsightly. . . .
>
> The cure does not consist in generating flesh there, but in bringing it from a neighbouring part; this, when the change is inconsiderable, may lead to no loss of structure, and thus escape notice; when considerable, it cannot fail to be observed. . . .
>
> The following is the method of cure: first to reduce the mutilated part to a square; from its inner angles to make two transverse incisions turned towards the wound, so as completely to divide the part which lies within these lines from that beyond them; and afterwards, to approximate the part we have thus opened. If they do not completely meet, then, beyond these lines already made, we must make two lunar incisions turned towards the wound, so as to separate the integument only: for in this way its approximation will be facilitated: not that we are to use violence, but to gently draw it so that it may easily yield, and not retract considerably when let go. . . . Hence we are not to attempt to draw any thing either from the lower part of the ears, or from the middle of the nose [the lateral nasal cartilage], or the inferior parts of the nostrils [the ala], or from the angles of the lips. We may derive our supply from both sides when there is any defect at the summit or lower parts of the ears, the middle of the nose or nostrils, or in the centre of the lips. . . . Then, the approximated edges are to be sewed together, including the skin on both sides, and extending the suture to the lines above mentioned. . . . [M]ost commonly it becomes agglutinated on the seventh day. We are then to remove the sutures, and to complete the healing of the ulcers.[1]

Celsus is quite aware of the procedure's limits. One may say that his technique belongs to generalist practice. It is not until the Renaissance that a properly reconstructive intention appears, the project, that is, of reconstructive surgery, capable of treating mutilations that are more severe than those discussed by Celsus. Tagliacozzi's *De curtorum chirurgia per insitionem libri duo* [*Two Books on Graft Surgery on the Mutilated*] appears in Venice in 1597. The surgical procedure is modeled on the art of grafting. It is thus possible to draw lessons for the repair of wounds from the care of plants,

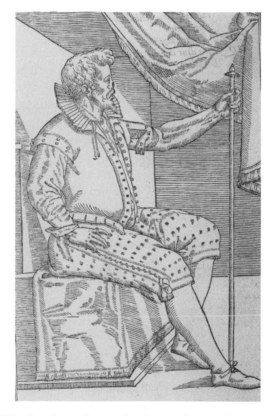

FIGURE 2-1. This plate shows the mutilated nose, the arm flap, and the area just underneath it. (Gaspare Tagliacozzi, *De curtorum chirurgia per insitionem* (Venice: Bindoni, 1597], plate V. Courtesy of Bibliothèque interuniversitaire de santé, Paris.)

and we know for example that the term *insitio*, graft, is used for the repair of wounds. Yet there is a fundamental difference between the activity of the surgeon and that of the gardener. The graft of a skin flap is a much more complicated operation than the graft of a branch because the part to be transplanted must be a fit both in structure and in form. The several phases of the operation are delicate. The skin flap to be grafted has to be prepared and then be inserted into the part to be repaired. When the graft has taken, the parts must carefully be kept together throughout the scarring process. Then the excised tissue of the arm flap must be separated from its initial place. Finally, the grafted part must be given the form of a nose, and for the result to last, care must be taken to avoid complications.

Tagliacozzi provides a clear exposition of his surgical technique:

> Because lips, nose, and ears are made of skin (which cannot sprout anew, so to speak, once it is cut away), the founders of our art established the practice of grafting skin from another location in order to restore the dignity of the injured part. Moreover, no part of the body can be more safely and effortlessly removed and transplanted than skin. . . . The graft must . . . be taken from a part of the body that is rarely seen unclothed. The most important consideration in this matter is that the operation involve as little danger as possible. That the upper arm meets these requirements admirably, and that there is no other part of the body so well suited to this operation, will soon become clear. The skin of the upper arm is very similar to that of the lips and nose. In addition, the inner aspect of the upper arm is hardly ever visible, and it offers a generous supply of skin that is especially suitable for repairing mutilations.[2]

A little further, Tagliacozzi asks the question whether the graft is to be taken from the patient or from someone else:

> The skin flap can, in fact, be procured from another person's body, which we can prove by appealing both to the ancient authorities and to reason. If we consider the strength of man's native heat as well as the natures and similarities of human temperaments, we will realize that there is no reason why the graft should not, without any difficulty, be taken from the body of another. . . . Cato tells us that plants of the same type can be grafted, as in his example of joining an inferior scion to a nobler stock. Columella, moreover, demonstrates that even the grafting of different types of trees, such as the

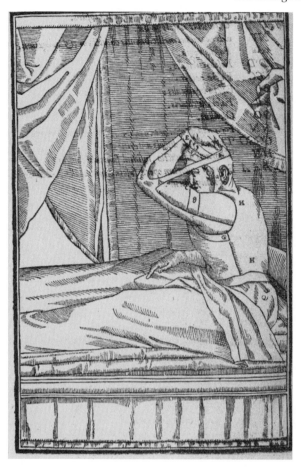

FIGURE 2-2. This plate shows the posterior part and left side of the bandage during the immobilization phase. (Gaspare Tagliacozzi, *De curtorum chirurgia per insitionem* [Venice: Bindoni, 1597], plate IX. Courtesy of Bibliothèque interuniversitaire de santé, Paris.)

olive and the fig, can be successful. Why, then, should it be surprising that the skin of one person can serve as a graft for another? . . . If the physician attempted to take the graft from a person other than the patient, the outcome would surely be imperiled. The skin flap must be firmly sutured to the mutilated nose or lips until the parts coalesce; moreover, we must restrict its

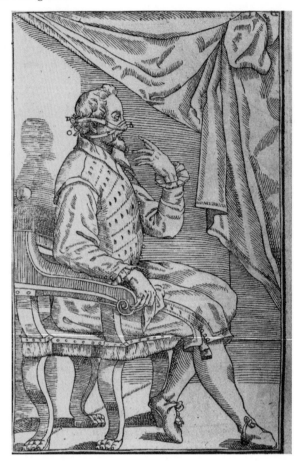

FIGURE 2-3. By the bandage around the nose, this plate shows the anticipation of the nose's modeling. (Gaspare Tagliacozzi, *De curtorum chirurgia per insitionem* [Venice: Bindoni, 1597], plate XI. Courtesy of Bibliothèque interuniversitaire de santé, Paris.)

motion as much as possible lest the delicate union be weakened. Would two people ever consent to being bound together so intimately and for so long? I certainly cannot imagine it. How could the physician ensure the survival of the graft? How difficult it would be for the parties involved to eat, sleep, sit, stand, or perform any other necessary actions![3]

At the end of the eighteenth century, the English discover a method of repairing noses long practiced by Hindus. Military doctors describe the Indian method in the *Madras Gazette* as early as 1792. In 1794 the *Gentleman's Magazine* publishes an article in the form of a letter from a certain B. L. addressed to the editor Sylvanus Urban that contains a description and detailed drawing of a surgical reconstruction of the nose, operated on an Indian named Cowasjee, who has worked as bullock-driver in the English army during the Third Anglo-Mysore War. Captured by Tipu Sultan, he

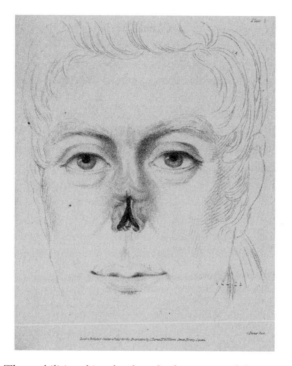

FIGURE 2-4. The syphilitic subject has lost the front parts of the nose, with the exception of a small portion of the *alae* or the sides of the nostrils. (Joseph Constantine Carpue, *An Account of Two Successful Operations for Restoring a Lost Nose From the Integuments of the Forehead* [etc.] [London: Longman, Hurst, Rees, Orme and Brown, 1816], no pagination. Courtesy of Bibliothèque interuniversitaire de santé, Paris.)

has had his nose and one hand cut off. Having rejoined the Bombay Army, he remains twelve months without a nose, after which period he is successfully operated on "by a man of the Brickmaker cast" near Pune.

The following technique is used:

> A thin plate of wax is fitted to the stump of the nose, so as to make a nose of good appearance. It is then flattened, and laid on the forehead. A line is drawn around the wax, and the operator then dissects off as much skin as it covered, leaving undivided a small slip between the eyes. This slip preserves the circulation till an union has taken place between the new and old parts. The cicatrix of the stump of the nose is then pared off, and immediately behind this raw part an incision is made through the skin, which passes around both *alæ*, and goes along the upper lip. The skin is now brought down from the forehead, and, being twisted half round, its edge is inserted into this incision, so that a nose is formed with a double hold above, and with its *alæ* and *septum* below fixed in the incision. A little *Terra Japonica* is softened with water, and being spread on slips of cloth, five or six of these are placed over each other, to secure the joining. No other dressing but this cement is used for four days. It is then removed, and cloths dipped in ghee (a kind of butter) are applied. The connecting slips of skin are divided about the 25th day, when a little more dissection is necessary to improve the appearance of the new nose. For five or six days after the operation, the patient is made to lie on his back; and, on the tenth day, bits of soft cloth are put into the nostrils to keep them sufficiently open. This operation is very generally successful. The artificial nose is secure, and looks nearly as well as the natural one; nor is the scar on the forehead very observable after a length of time.[4]

The discovery of the Indian method leads to the recuperation of the Italian method and to new applications. Sprengel gives us the narrative of these first attempts at rhinoplasty:

> After he had much practiced on corpses, J. C. Carpue in 1814 conducted the first [Indian nose construction] on a man who had lost the tip, septum and cartilage of the nose to mercurial disease. Just like the Hindus he fitted a waxen model to the stump, and traced around this a line to designate the area to scarify; then, after cleanly having shaved off the hair on the forehead, he flattened the model, inversed it, placed it on the forehead and traced around it the flap to be cut out. He now scarified the stump of the nose, made a

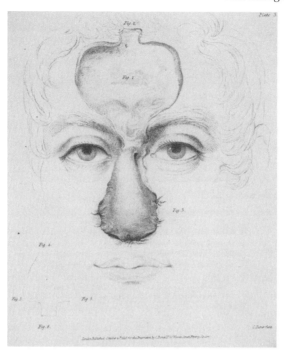

FIGURE 2-5. The state of the nose and the wound on the forehead as they appear after surgery. Figures 4 and 5 depict the *alae*, 6 the septum of the nose. (Joseph Constantine Carpue, *An Account of Two Successful Operations for Restoring a Lost Nose From the Integuments of the Forehead* [etc.] [London: Longman, Hurst, Rees, Orme and Brown, 1816], 88. Courtesy of Bibliothèque interuniversitaire de santé, Paris.)

simple lateral cut for the septum at the upper lip, separated the traced-out forehead flap from the pericranium, turned it out, brought septum and lateral parts into proper contact, and affixed them with sutures and patches; the wound on the forehead, however, he sought to tighten as much as possible. On the third day already, the union had taken place, but the new nose was entirely flat and rose at every breath. On the sixth day, he removed all sutures; a mistake made in the diet caused a small separation at the *alea* that he, however, reattached, and in the fourth month, finally, he cut through the skin fold at the root of the nose and united the parts with sutures thanks to which, he tells us, a rather natural nose had been produced. . . . Even before

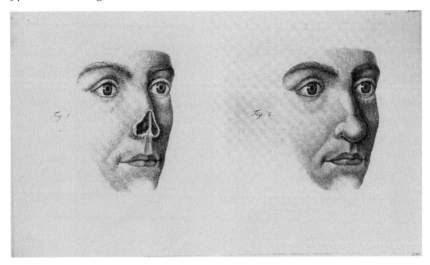

FIGURE 2-6. Reparation of a mutilation of the nose. (Carl Ferdinand von Gräfe, *Rhinoplastik oder die Kunst den Verlust der Nase organisch zu ersetzen* [Berlin: Realschulbuchhandlung, 1818], plate 3. Courtesy of Bibliothèque interuniversitaire de santé, Paris.)

> Carpue's work had become known in Germany, C. F. Gräfe had performed
> the procedure according to Tagliacozzi in Berlin in 1816 . . . Gräfe rightly
> criticized Tagliacozzi's method for its protraction and the Indian method for
> the new deformity caused by its scarring of the forehead, and he sought to
> improve the first method mainly by affixing the arm flap to the stump of the
> nose immediately after it had been cut out without waiting for its protracted
> cicatrization, as Reneaulme had suggested long before: an improvement
> which he then named the German Method and according to which he and
> several of his students have successfully operated.[5]

The importation of the Indian method to England has two consequences. The first is of a practical kind, the testing of forehead flap techniques and, not without modifications, of arm flap techniques. No one doubts that these therapeutic acts mark the renewal of reconstructive surgery. The second consequence concerns a historical point, the reasons given by Carpue and his contemporaries for the occultation of Tagliacozzi's work. I have to dwell

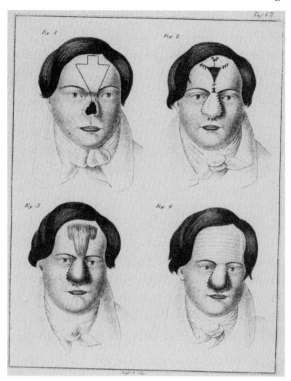

FIGURE 2-7. The Indian forehead flap method. (Hermann Eduard Fritze and
O. F. G. Reich, *Die plastische Chirurgie* [Berlin: Hirschwald, 1845], § 63, plate VII.
Courtesy of Bibliothèque interuniversitaire de santé, Paris.)

for a moment on their versions of history, show their fragility and capture
their significance.

Different Versions of History

Very soon, Carpue and his contemporaries related the renascence of reconstructive surgery to the discovery of the Indian method. From there, the
very first look taken at the history of this surgical specialty was a look back at

Tagliacozzi's *De curtorum chirurgica*. It is well known that Andreas Vesalius's 1543 *De humani corporis fabrica* [*On the Fabric of the Human Body*] enjoyed an immediate, striking, and enduring renaissance. Curiously, the same cannot be said for the fabrication of noses. Despite the close connections that tie surgery and anatomy to one another, the disciplines do not share the same spirit. Surgery repairs, restores, and unites what anatomy separates, undoes, and isolates. Learned dissections precede the dissolution of flesh. Surgery attempts to undo the wounds of the flesh. The most profound difference, perhaps, is this: the fabric of the body shows the organs that make up the body while the fabrication of the nose explains how to restore it. Anatomy dismantles the parts of the body. It is the analysis of an organic totality. Nose surgery aims at the reconstitution of an organic part in its totality. Therapeutic practices, unlike anatomy, are perfectible. Of course anatomy did not emerge all complete from the hands of the first anatomists. I would just like to underscore this epistemological fact: throughout its history, surgical practice, unlike dissection procedures, has never stopped reforming itself. One question, however, remains unanswered: Why was Tagliacozzi's procedure ignored for so long? Certainly, the Enlightenment was indifferent to the central question of the repair of noses. We must say *central* because "good old Musitano liked a beautiful nose."[6] For him, this organ was like the sun of the face, its most beautiful ornament. And yet the Tagliacozzi's erudite, astonishing work must be understood as the manual *par excellence* of nose restoration. Why was this great book neglected? To this phenomenon, Carpue and his contemporaries ascribe a certain number of causes.

As far as motives are concerned, the first they name is the injury's exceptional character. If mutilations of the nose had been accidents as banal as breaking a bone, surgeons would quickly have gotten to work on the problems posed by the injury: "The paucity of cases is the principal feature to be regarded. Had the loss of a nose been as frequent as the fracture of a limb, the treatment of the first accident would have been as anxiously provided for as the second."[7] Tagliacozzi's art could have become part of the history of reconstructive surgery, but only as a pioneering attempt and under one condition, namely that reconstructive surgery itself have a history—which is not at all the case. In fact, the last stage, represented so well by the operation performed by the German surgeon Gräfe, is but a reactualization of the initial operation. In a word, Tagliacozzi's technique of repairing noses disappears along with its inventor. And when it reappears two centuries later, it is almost identical to how it was conceived and put into practice by him.

This first explanation forms part of a medical imaginary. It is curious to see how Carpue accounts for the abandonment of the technique. He invokes the absence of practice, due to a lack of cases. He opposes the exception (the mutilation of noses) to the rule (the breaking of limbs). That is where the error lies: Carpue forgets that these injuries necessitate therapeutic acts that cannot be compared: here the immobilization of a broken bone, there the compensation for a lack by means of an autotransplant. The art of correcting a fracture by means of reduction differs from the art of correcting by means of a graft the way an art that borrows from mechanics differs from the art of gardening. To play the exception off against the rule, it is necessary to confuse skin and bones or the exterior and the frame. It is necessary to place skin grafts and repairs of bone fractures on the same level. Carpue would be more inspired if he compared the mutilation of noses to the amputation of limbs. To hide a mutilation, the physician can fit an artificial nose just as he replaces a cut-off hand with a prosthesis. Provided he reasons as a practitioner of transplants, he would confront the same obstacle: a missing nose cannot be replaced by another nose any more than a cut-off hand can be replaced with another.

Carpue's is a curious way of accounting for how a major work is forgotten. On his reading, since the pathology did not exist, it was normal for nobody to be interested in it. As a result, the occultation of *De curtorum chirurgia* cannot be ascribed to any blinding on the part of surgeons whatsoever. It would be wrong to regard as negligence what is, quite simply, inexperience: The absence of patients is what has kept surgeons from applying their talents, refining the method and recognizing the value of Tagliacozzi's procedure. Strictly speaking, rhinoplasty has no history because it has not existed as a medical specialty. Tagliacozzi's name is the sign of a nonevent.

The second reason, which complements the first, is a cultural reason. To affirm that reconstructive surgery did not exist for lack of cases amounts to saying that it did not exist for lack of cut-off noses. In Europe, it is not habitual to cut off noses. This rather barbaric punitive practice simply is not as current in our highly civilized countries. Carpue underscores this point:

"It is to be doubted, whether, even in the time of Taliacotius, the number of cases requiring the assistance of the art was equal, in the west of Europe, to the number in the east; in countries bordering on Asiatic and African nations, and tinged with their manners."[8]

In fact, however, the mutilation of noses was far from being confined to exceptional accidents: the cut-off nose was a common injury in Europe. There are multiple occasions for its occurrence: wars, duels, fights. Severe mutilation, which renders people unrecognizable, is a procedure of exclusion. The individual thus marked is chased from the community. Mutilation is also a punitive procedure. To expose visible, indelible marks is to take vengeance for an offence or to punish an abuse. Mutilation stigmatizes, humiliates, and degrades: it is a punishment of choice. Dionis gives a good example: Disfiguration is at the same time the right kind of vengeance and the right kind of verdict. The Paris Parliament condemns a notary's wife for having cut off the nose of her husband's mistress. Yet the judges invented a new ordeal for the notary's wife. They sentence her to having a *fleur-de-lis* burnt into her forehead with a hot iron. But the king, who finds this judgment to be too cruel, pardons her. Women thus cut off their husbands' mistresses' noses, or their husbands' noses, as if, to use Musitano's phrase, "this body part was to endure the punishment for a crime of which it was innocent, this part and not a certain other that alone was guilty."[9] There is no dearth of cut-off noses in Europe. Nor is there a judicial void. In the seventeenth century, the Paris Parliament decides that the nose is a limb and that from then on out it is to be considered as such in matters of criminal jurisprudence. And, concluding on the affective register, I must mention self-mutilation, the disfiguration that provokes repulsion. In England, women cut off their noses to dissuade Danish invaders from raping them. The abbess of the monastery of St. Cyr in Marseille does the same to preserve her virginity as the Saracens approached: "A courageous action," according to Muralt, "that was imitated by her forty nuns and that so outraged the ferocious conquerors that they killed them all."[10]

To note what is essential here: to say that mutilation as punishment was not current in Europe is to reinforce the idea that occasions for repair did not exist. There are no noses to repair because there is no reason to cut them off. No injury whatsoever allows surgeons to focus their attention on how to heal them. The injury occurring so rarely, it is normal that no one has any knowledge of or experience with it. Once more, it is not an indifference or lack of inventiveness that is at issue; the scarcity of cut-off noses explains everything.

The third, sociological, reason is in line with the preceding two. It accounts for the lack of interest in Tagliacozzi's method. For those who rediscover the Bologna physician's work, it is as if Southern Italy was an enclave of barbarism in civilized Europe. Tagliacozzi's practice flourishes in a place that offers a clientele of crooks with cut-off noses: traitors, womanizers, adventurers, and thieves. The forehead flap technique, on this reading, first makes it to Italy by way of the Arabs, who have themselves adopted it from the Hindus. But there's more: a modification of the procedure that takes local custom into account. In Sicily and Calabria, the extraction of skin according to the Indian method leaves a mark on the forehead that is perceived as degrading. The smallest scar in this area becomes suspect since it is common to leave a withering mark there with a red-hot iron to punish shameful and dishonoring crimes. If the operation that consists in covering up the sign of one infamy (the cut-off nose) provokes another (the mark on the forehead), it is without benefit. It is thus necessary to extract the skin flap from a less-exposed part of the body. The arm flap procedure thus appears as the ultimate avatar of the Indian technique: a local variant well adapted to Sicilian customs; a practice of choice for wicked men; a practice, in any case, that does not leave a scar on the forehead.

This version, appealing though it may be, is historically wrong. One would be wrong to think of the arm flap technique as a practice of conjurers adept at covering up the outcome of some sort of fraud. Without a doubt, the families of surgeons in Southern Italy have kept this solid tradition of reconstructive surgery alive. Tagliacozzi is aware of their technique; he has read Fioravanti, which might be the reason why he dedicates his life to the reconstructive surgery of the nose. Tagliacozzi cites his predecessors: Alessandro Benedetti and Gustavo Branca. But he also criticizes them for not having described the operation, for maintaining a culture of secrets. Tagliacozzi is a modern man. He does not present himself as the inventor of the autotransplant technique but as the one who has pushed it as far as possible, just as he reveals it to his readers. Tagliacozzi has also given this popular practice the status of an academic discipline. In addition, his art has become synonymous with a rare and fancy procedure for the well-to-do. His procedure, thanks to its complexity, its precision, and its ritual is out of sync with its time, a luxury within the reach of aristocrats alone.

By underlining the popular origin of the procedure, Carpue, Pierre-François Percy and Charles Nicolas Laurent disparage both the man and the surgical specialty. They disparage the man because Tagliacozzi is trapped in a history that knows no ruptures: if he has predecessors, not only is he not the inventor of the procedure, he also appears as the debtor of the Branca and Vianeo families. He appears simply to be a compiler, a usurper, even:

> The restoration in question was known, even common, when Tagliacozzi usurped it to talk about it lengthily, heavily, boringly. Yet we are obliged to this writer for having collected and preserved some good traditions and for having converted them into a corpus of doctrines—not according to his own experience, since we are led to believe that he never redid a single nose, but according to the true hands-on experiences of men like the Boiani, the Brancas, Pavone, Montigore.[11]

The more Tagliacozzi's art is marked by its regional origins, the more this surgical specialty is devalued. Put differently, if the practice Tagliacozzi promotes has been anchored in Sicilian folklore for a long time, it can in no way lay claim to the dignity of a therapeutic method. The repair of noses does not have a place in the surgical arts.

The forth and last reason invoked to explain the oblivion into which Tagliacozzi has fallen is the series of inconveniences the technique brings with it. The intervention associates a procedure from advanced surgery and an autotransplant. Yet the transplant has to take into account the constraints imposed by the biological time necessary for the preparation of the arm flap and for the transplant. Critics underline how arduous and confining the procedure was. The patient has to remain immobile in an uncomfortable position for several weeks, even months.

The posture the patient has to take in the fixation apparatus certainly is impressive. In the end, this image might have exercised a dissuasive function. The patient becomes a tortured man, a fiction so deplorable that it has been affirmed, for example by Percy and Laurent, that Tagliacozzi never performed such an operation. It goes so far that all the objections once raised by Vesalius, Gabriele Falloppio, and Ambroise Paré are once again brought up against Tagliacozzi, without much concern for the fact that these criticisms were aimed not at Tagliacozzi but his Sicilian or Calabrian predecessors or for the fact that Tagliacozzi had carefully taken precautions against such an amalgam, likely to discredit his technique. Vesalius and the others speak of what has been known for a long time, though only by hearsay. They say the patient has to plunge what remains of his nose into the live flesh of his arm until it grows and forms a sort of nose. They say that this portion of the procedure is painful and cruel and that the patient needs to remain motionless for forty days, even for several months. In his letter to Girolamo Mercuriale, published in 1587 in the second edition of *De decoratione*, Tagliacozzi brushes aside all these inanities: not only does the operation consist in attaching an arm flap to the stump, it is also well-tolerated and the immobilization time does not exceed two weeks.

The Indian method is discovered at the turn of the eighteenth and nineteenth centuries and makes the repair of the nose possible. It also makes it necessary to marshal a fictive history in which Tagliacozzi's procedure is far from offering the same advantages. Here lies the origin of the ascription of the procedure's abandonment to its strangeness, its cruel refinement even. In essence, this is an underhanded promotion campaign for a lucrative deal, and Tagliacozzi serves as whipping boy for an advertising campaign. Percy and Laurent are latecomers: they reason like Falloppio who advised Tycho Brahe to opt for a fake nose instead of difficult surgery. But they are business-savvy: they offer a cardboard nose and glasses of their own design, a cheap nose available for purchase at Marassi and Chol, mask makers in the rue Bourg-l'Abbé:

> We are tempted to think that it would be to pay too dearly for a reproduction that is almost always misshapen and that it would be better for everyone to keep to the kind of artificial piece we will talk about because, well executed, it brings together the advantages of great resemblance and perfect illusion, the convenience of use and wear, the fact that it costs but little in money and nothing in suffering. It is an artificial nose, of which I have commissioned a drawing that is included at the end of this article.[12]

In the history of medicine, such historical reconstructions serve as retrospective justifications. If physicians have had so many good reasons not to follow the path opened by Tagliacozzi, it would be inappropriate to reproach them for it, since what should be viewed exclusively in relation to the limits of Tagliacozzi's technique would have to be put down to the scarcity of cases or to a cruel practice. In fact, however, we need to reverse the order of factors: the method is neglected not because the cases are rare but because the conditions of its application are exceptional. The operation is singular in more than one respect. It does not really aim at producing a beautiful nose. It has to compensate a lack without, however, repudiating the restoration of a graceful form. The deformity to be repaired (an old injury) does not, after all, call for an active, immediate cure, the surgeon's habitual lot. But there's more: considering the material conditions of possibility of its application, the procedure applies only to the rich.

It still happens today that Tagliacozzi is hardly understood any better. Very recently, Professor Bertrand pointed out that since in the case of Tagliacozzi's procedure one should speak of "rhinopoesis," it would be wrong to inscribe Tagliacozzi's procedure in a history of rhinoplasty. But is rhinopoesis by means of skin flaps not synonymous with rhinoplasty by means of autoplasty? And since Professor Bertrand is not to be suspected of pedantry, we need to find out where the difference lies for him. I can see only one answer: rhinopoesis consists in making a nose with the help of a skin flap while rhinoplasty is an operation of facial sculpting. The fabrication of a nose is not to be confused with the modification of its form.

This erudite distinction raises two questions. Can there be *rhinopoesis*, that is to say, reconstruction of noses, without surgeons' concerning themselves with their form? On this point, Tagliacozzi is so meticulous that he applies a sort of mask to his patients. Does he not dream of creating forms by simple molding? The result could no doubt be but an approximation. It is quite possible that this is simply, to take up Professor Bertrand's catchy expression, "shaping a potato." From this point of view, it is easier to understand the reservations about the use of the term *rhinoplasty*: one should not confuse a rather coarse attempt at reconstruction with the prowess of plastic surgery.

But can one qualify a procedure this old on the basis of a retrospective judgment of its results? The answer to this question has to be no. When it comes to the demands of form, the result (potato or not) is of little importance. It would be an anachronism to speak of *rhinopoesis* to name an operation for which the surgeons who discovered it had already coined the term *rhinoplasty*. Carl Ferdinand von Gräfe, who follows in Tagliacozzi's footsteps, is the first to use the term in his 1818 book, *Rhinoplastik, oder die Kunst den Verlust der Nase organisch zu ersetzen [Rhinoplasty, or the Art of Compensating Organically for the Loss of a Nose]*. Ten years later, the words *rhinoplasty* and *rhinoplastics* appear in the *Encyclopédie méthodique [Methodical Encyclopedia]*: "Surgical operation by which the difformity that results from a loss of the nose is cured. Rhinoplasty has been known in Europe for no more than three hundred years, but authentic accounts lead us to believe that it has been in use since time immemorial among certain peoples of the Indies where the mutilation of the nose is a very common punishment."[13]

A Latency Period

One might object that subsequent historians of medicine have not made the same mistakes as their predecessors; they enjoy more latitude than those who discovered the Indian method to such astonishment. Very recently, Paolo Santoni-Rugiu and Philip J. Sykes have presented an exhaustive and erudite chapter of the history of nasal reconstruction in their great 2007 book, *History of Plastic Surgery*. In the section they entitle "The decline of rhinoplasty," the authors recall the motifs that they say contributed to the occultation of Tagliacozzi's technique. They insist on the limited number of copies of the first edition of *De curtorum chirurgia*, followed by the death of the author: "If Tagliacozzi had lived longer, his continued surgical and teaching activities would surely have contributed to the spread of his method." They also underscore the resistance Tagliacozzi's art allegedly encountered:

> The attitude of the Church, even if its past interdictions were no longer formally observed, continued to pose an obstacle to the acceptance of modern surgical methods. . . . There is no question that in ecclesiastical circles there was opposition to surgery and this existed even in the relatively enlightened University of Bologna. In . . . Tagliacozzi's case the specific accusation that he had acted against the will of God led to his exclusion, however briefly, from burial in consecrated ground.

Following Joseph G. McCarthy, finally, they invoke a reason that is of the order of epistemology:

> The end of the sixteenth century witnessed a decline in the art of surgery all over Europe, and Italy was no exception, despite the significant discoveries that were being made in other fields of medicine by such figures as Vesalius, Redi and Bellini. J. G. McCarthy has written that "ironically the Age of Enlightenment was not the Age of Enlightenment for plastic surgery." This period of obscurantism continued well into the seventeenth century and certainly did nothing to encourage the spread of Tagliacozzi's teachings.[14]

This version is historically false. It is true that Tagliacozzi dies relatively young. But his death does not prevent his work from being known and disseminated, thanks to some pirated and several reeditions. Tagliacozzi's art is part of the medical field, without religious contestation. The short episode of his exclusion from the cemetery where he has been buried has to be put down to a conspiracy. The Inquisition tribunal quickly recognizes that the accusations of which he is the victim are based on lies. Four years later, his remains are placed in a sepulcher in the cloister of San Giovanni Batista in Bologna. As early as 1582 he receives an homage engraved in stone, "Gaspare Tagliacozzi, man of genius and of science, skilled anatomist."[15] Later, a statue is erected in his honor in the anatomical theater of Bologna University, which shows him holding a nose in his left hand.[16] Why does the majority of historians of surgery paint the Enlightenment in the colors of the Middle Ages? The answer, perhaps, can be found in the most recent past of aesthetic facial surgery. In 1933 Raymond Passot begins the first chapter of his book, *Sculptor of Faces*, with the words: "Despite all the obstacles placed in its way, despite the mockery of the skeptics, the criticisms of the ill-wishers, one thing cannot be denied: the prodigious development of aesthetics over the last ten years."[17] It is quite possible that this reputation of a disliked specialty is projected on the history of its beginnings. Due to a desire that the birth of the young discipline of aesthetic surgery be marked by a victory over its detractors, Tagliacozzi already has to face a dark plot.

But chronology is not subject to modification. Tagliacozzi publishes his work without facing the slightest epistemological, religious or moral contestation. Yet Carpue and his contemporaries have the feeling they are

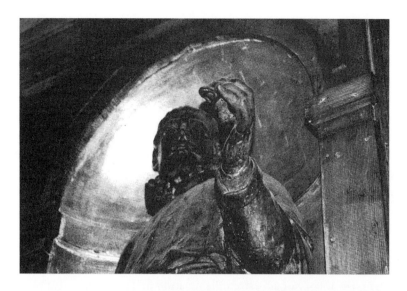

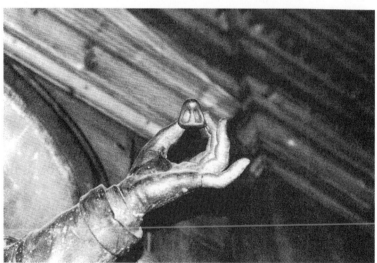

FIGURE 2-8. (*Top*) Statue of Gaspare Tagliacozzi (1545–99), sculpted in 1734 by Silvestro Giannotti, two detail views. It was restored after having been damaged during bombing in 1944. It stands in the anatomical theater of the University of Bologna, built in 1637 by the architect Antonio Levanti. (Bottom) Detail: Statue of Gaspare Tagliacozzi. (Photo courtesy of Biblioteca Comunale dell'Archginnasio, Bologna.)

rediscovering his procedure. A latency period separates Tagliacozzi's text from its rediscovery at the turn of the eighteenth and nineteenth centuries, two centuries during which several systems of thought intersect to constitute a framework whose autonomy and solidity exclude the memory of Tagliacozzi's art. On the one hand, his procedure is perceived as an extraordinary case of transplantation because the technique of the autograft of an arm flap is confused with a nose transplant. On the other, there is ridicule of the Royal Society's virtuoso activities. The story of a nose graft with a donor seems like a choice target. In the eyes of the mockers, the procedure is a mystification. Later, throughout the eighteenth century, we see innovative research on grafts and transplants. The manipulation of living organisms passes into the hands of experimenters; hence the invention of animal chimera. They quickly encourage new surgical practices, like the immediate reimplantation of cut-off noses, and do so all the more quickly as at this very moment, the theory of adhesive inflammation finds a privileged application in cases of mutilation. The field of immediate healing, theoretical and empirical at the same time, is constituted in the Enlightenment. It is theoretical because surgical practice is undergirded by a theory of injury formation. It is empirical to the extent to which surgical practice is founded on a sort of primitive autoplasty. This is the point at which repression happens: the act of rapid replantation is foreign to so complex a procedure as Tagliacozzi's repairs. Tagliacozzi practices a sort of secondary autoplasty quite a long time after the scarring of the wound. The preeminence of reconstructive surgery has not made it possible to understand Tagliacozzi's lesson. It is one thing to recuperate one's nose, to bring it back to oneself or to enter into its possession. It is quite another thing to have a nose fabricated or reformed all in one piece. But let's not get ahead of ourselves.

It is Elisio Calenzio who, by talking of an extraordinary transplant, discounts the arm flap procedure in advance. The first reference to a nose graft with a donor can be found in his 1558 letter to Orpianus: "If you would like to have your nose repaired, come see me in Italy. Truly, the thing is a marvel among men. Branca, a man of genius and skill, has learnt to graft on noses by either taking part of the arm or by borrowing one from a slave."[18] From the beginning of the seventeenth century on, the arm flap technique disappears in favor of an astonishing procedure. Tagliagozzi is credited with being a father of a nose transplant he has never performed. This organ transplant is also inserted into the framework of a vitalist medical philosophy. Van Helmont tells a strange story. It is the story of a Brussels nobleman who, out of fear of the arm flap graft procedure, prefers to have the nose of a peasant from the Bologna countryside grafted onto his face—against payment:

> After about 13. moneths after his returne to his owne countrey, on a suddaine the ingrafted nose grew cold, putrified, and within few dayes, dropt off. To those of his friends, that were curious in the exploration of the cause of this unexpected misfortune, it was discovered, that the Porter expired, neer about the same punctilio of time, wherein the nose grew frigid and cadaverous. There are at *Bruxels* yet surviving, some of good repute, that were eye-witnesses of these occurrences. Is not this *Magnetisme* of manifest affinity with *mumie*, whereby the nose, enjoying, by title and right of inoculation, a community of life, sense and vegetation, for so many moneths, on a suddaine mortified on the other side of the Alpes? I pray, what is there in this of Superstition? what of attent and exalted *Imagination*?[19]

To understand this story, one must specify the meaning of some concepts endowed with great powers. They belong to a philosophy that dominated all of therapeutic medicine. Where does this idea of transplantation come from? To associate the malady with a plant, it suffices at that time to identify the cause of a malady as some sort of seed. On the basis of medical ontology, Paracelsus imagined it to be possible to transport the sickness of one individual to another by having them live together. This procedure he called *morbid transplantation*. The aim is to heal a sick individual by carrying his sickness over into a healthy body. The concept *mumia* guarantees the connection, unity and solidarity of the organic parts thanks to which the procedure is destined to succeed. To be more precise one would have to say that actions at a distance guarantee the success of this practice, a magical practice whose finality it is to heal. The *mumia* names the portion of the vital spirit that is linked to blood, maintains the warmth of the parts and guarantees the cohesion of the organism, so many properties that it preserves even when it is separated from the body. It is understandable that, under these conditions, the *mumia* transplanted onto a recipient conserves an imperishable sympathy for the living being from which it is taken.

We can see immediately that if the malady consists in a mutilation, the therapeutic act must be symmetrical to and the inverse of the act that guarantees the cure by morbid transplantation. In homage to Paracelsus, we could call this *salutary transplantation*. In the case of the organ transplant, the remedy is of the body: it is a limb, an organic part taken from a living being. The Paracelsian principle is pushed to its extreme: after the nose is cut off the donor, its transplantation repairs the mutilation of the recipient. We know that after the separation of a part it may happen that it be reproduced—hence the restoration of the organic totality. This phenomenon of regeneration can be observed in the animal kingdom. But if the injury is lethal, an opposite phenomenon is observed: the dissolution of the living being in its totality. If the subject dies, in this case the donor, then his nose, which has been transplanted, also dies because it still clings to the whole from which it has been separated. That is why the Brussels nobleman's nose falls off. The concept *mumia* names a magnetic force that works across distances. It allows van Helmont to keep at bay the idea of enchantment, bewitchment even, which is so closely associated with the participation of Satan.

This story is certainly responsible for the substitution of the autograft procedure by the phantasm of the allograft with donor. We find variants of van Helmont's story in the writings of several physicians. Dionis, for example, takes up the tale of the autograft but this time with a—dare I say it—involuntary donor. His story suffices to show how the classical age could move so quickly from gross disdain to incredulity:

> We are not to think that it's possible to make a Nose which is wholly cut off to take again. But yet we are told that some Thieves having in the Night attack'd some Passengers, one of those Rogues receiv'd a cut on the Nose, which took it quite off, and that going to be dress'd, the Chirurgeon ask'd for his Nose, in order to sow it on if he had it; that his Comrades immediately run and cut off the Nose of a Man which they unluckily met with in the way, and bringing it to the Chirurgeon, he perform'd the Suture, by means of which that part was grafted on, and grew to that part of the Robber's Nose which was left, as a Graft would have done [to] a Tree.[20]

Very quickly, authors go as far as associating Tagliacozzi with the operation that consisted in the graft of a flap from a donor's gluteus. Butler finds in this new phantasm a choice subject to express his hatred of scholars. We know how in seventeenth-century England conservatives mock those who they derisively call *virtuosos*. Their sarcasms bear down on all who care a little too much for experimental philosophy. But what is said against science?

> That it inclines men to be unsetled, and *contentious*; That it takes up more of their time, than men of business ought to bestow; That it makes them *Romantic*, and subject to frame more perfect images of things, than the things themselves will bear; That it renders them overweening, unchangeable, and obstinat; That thereby men become averse from a practical cours, and unable to bear the difficulties of action; That it emploies them about things, which are no where in use in the world; and, That it draws them to neglect and contemn their own present times, by doting on the past.[21]

In *Gulliver's Travels*, Jonathan Swift describes the Academy of Lagado, where emaciated scholars torture dogs to death by breathing air into the posterior orifice. Butler cannot do with less. In this way, Tagliacozzi finds himself in the company of useless men: Boyle, Hooke, Lower, Mayow, and Willis. Within the framework of this demolition of nascent scientific rationality, the nose graft becomes an object of sarcasm. The procedure spitefully attributed to Tagliacozzi joins the fantasies of the disciples of experimental science.

> So learned Taliacotius from
> The brawny part of Porter's Bum,
> Cut supplemental Noses, which
> Would last as long as Parent Breech:
> But when the Date of Nock was out,
> Off dropt the Sympathetick Snout.[22]

In the middle of the eighteenth century, Voltaire takes up the torch. He is all too willing to conceive of a partial allograft of the face, but only to ridicule it: "Taliacotius, the great Etrurian Aesculap, . . . craftily took a piece of a poor man's ass, and properly adjusted it to the nose . . . Finally, it happened that just at the death of the donor the nose of the recipient fell off. And one often placed the nose in the same coffin, according to the dead man's wish and as a matter of justice and consensus, next to his behind."[23]

The final avatar of the gluteus flap: In the nineteenth century, there is serious discussion of a variant of the Indian method that uses the skin of the gluteus to redo the nose. With the exception of Butler's, or Voltaire's, high poetry, the search for the slightest trace of this variant in the medical literature would be in vain. Paul Bert, in his 1863 medical dissertation *De la greffe animale* [*On the Animal Graft*], seems to smell the rat.

But we should not believe that only the literary types crave this sort of fictions. Dionis does not hesitate to transfer onto Tagliacozzi all the criticisms that Paré, Gourmelin, and Fallappio already, and wrongly, level at the Calabrian surgeons. From incredulity to this amalgam, the circle is complete:

> 'Tis also storied of a Chirurgeon, that he made an Incision in the Arm of a Man who had just had his Nose cut off, that he clapp'd the Bloody part of the Nose into the Incision, and by a Bandage kept it some time in that posture; and that the Nose being stuck to the Flesh of the Arm, the Operator cut out as much of it as was requisite to shape a Nose, and that by this Operation he substituted another in the Place of that which was lost. But I take these Stories to be Apocryphal, and to be invented rather for Diversion, than to be real Truths.[24]

In the eighteenth century, the questions that concern the transplantation of body parts are developed on an unprecedented scale. The research of Duhamel du Monceau and Hunter testifies directly to this development. Duhamel du Monceau places a spur on the head of a cock:

> Here we have an organized part that has been detached from a cock's claw when it was no bigger than a grain of hempseed and which, having been placed on the head of that same animal, developed a rather intimate union and grew to several inches in length, conserving in this place the same organization it had in its original place, except that here it has become larger. One must agree that this truly is a graft practiced on an animal.[25]

As for Hunter, he repeats Duhamel du Monceau's experiments and confirms their results. He also inserts a freshly extracted human tooth in a rooster's comb. It looks as if a union has been operated between the comb and the blood vessels of the tooth. This method of grafting one part onto another is not limited to animals. It becomes a dentist's technique that Hunter publicizes: "Teeth, after having been drawn and inserted into the sockets of another person, unite to the new socket, which is called transplanting. Ingrafting and the inoculating of trees succeed upon the same principle."[26]

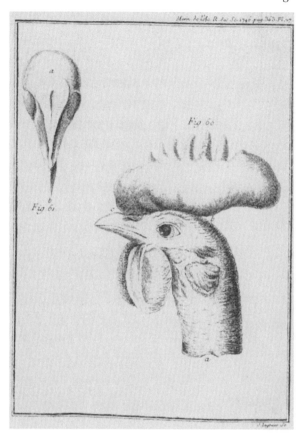

FIGURE 2-9. A rooster's head shown in its natural state to highlight the position of the comb (H. L. Duhamel du Monceau, "Recherches sur la reunion des plaies des arbres, sur la façon dont la greffe s'unit au sujet sur lequel on l'applique, sur la reunion des plaies des animaux, et quequels exemples de greffes appliqués sur des animaux," *Mémoire de l'Académie Royale des Sciences* [1746], 363, plate 27, figure 60. Courtesy of Bibliothèque interuniversitaire de santé, Paris.)

There is nothing in the nature of the cited facts to cast doubt on the good faith of those who cite them. Perhaps a certain number of these operations would have to have been presented, by conscientious researchers, in a more experimental fashion for medical thought to become less suspicious. Duhamel du Monceau and Hunter's experiments are not doubted;

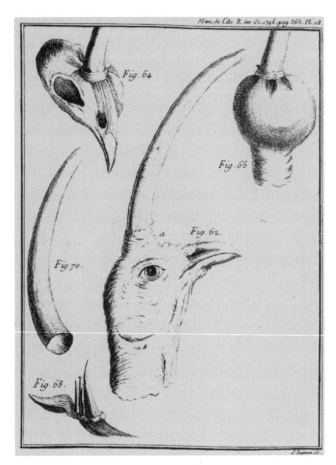

FIGURE 2-10. A rooster's head studded with a very large horn. (a) shows a cartilaginous ridge that rings its base. (Henri Louis Duhamel du Monceau, "Recherches sur la réunion des plaies des arbres, sur la façon dont la greffe s'unit au sujet sur lequel on l'applique, sur la réunion des plaies des animaux, et quelques exemples de greffes appliquées sur des animaux," 1746, *Mémoires de l'Académie des sciences* [Paris: Imprimerie royale, 1751], 363, plate 28, figure 62. Courtesy of Bibliothèque interuniversitaire de santé, Paris.)

why then would one doubt accounts in the same vein that are to be found in the medical literature? At first sight, these stories of noses cut off and replaced seemed improbable. In light of new animal grafts, they suddenly seemed credible; the first, unexpected, consequence of the experiments on the reunion of animal parts was the reactualization of accounts of cut-off noses being reimplanted on those who had lost them.

John Thomson cites some of these accounts:

> The first example of this kind which I find distinctly recorded is by Phio-
> ravant, in the 54th page of his second book of the Secrets of Surgery: "In
> that time, when I was in Africa," says Phioravant, "there happened a strange
> affair, and that was this:—A certain gentleman, a Spaniard, what was called
> Il Signior Andreas Gutiero, of the age of twenty-nine years, upon a time
> walked in the field, and fell at words with a soldier, and began to draw; the
> soldier seeing that, struck him with the left hand, and cut off his nose, and
> there it fell down in the sand. I then happened to stand by, and took it up,
> and pissed thereon to wash away the sand, and dressed it with our balsamo
> artificiato, and bound it up, and so left it to remain eight or ten days . . .
> when I did unbind it I found it fast conglutinated, and then I dressed it
> only once more, and he was perfectly whole, so that all Naples did wonder
> thereat, as is well known, for the said Signior Andreas doth live and can
> testify the same." Blegny, in his Zodiacus Medico Gallicus for the month
> of March 1680, mentions a case in which a nose that had been cut off with
> a sabre was replaced by a military surgeon of the name of Winsault, and in
> which a perfect reunion was obtained, he affirms, by the use of stiches [*sic*]
> and agglutinating plasters. . . .
>
> These are the only cases which I have been able to find distinctly stated
> of the re-union of a nose which had been completely cut off. This even, from
> analogy we have reason to believe, is possible, and nothing short of a con-
> trary testimony in the instances I have related, could justify us, I conceive, in
> denying the truth of the fact.[27]

The second consequence is in line with the first, more precisely, it is the practical complement or, rather, the actualization of the first. The graft of living parts from one animal to another has been the starting point for raising a new question in surgery. If it is possible to join body parts as un-like each other as comb and spur, it is *a forteriori* possible to rejoin a part separated from an organ by accident. Pouteau says there is infinitely less proximity between the spur and the comb than there is between the tip of the nose and the remainder of the nose. Garengeot describes a case not very different from those Thomson has found in the medical literature, the account of an operation that showed that a cut-off nose could be restored to its initial situation on the spot. In this case of a revivification of a separated nose by simple return of the nose to the lacuna of the mutilation, a soldier had been bitten in such a way that almost all of the nasal cartilage had been taken off:

> Sensing he had a piece of flesh in his mouth, his adversary spit it into the gutter and, all enraged, walked all over it as if to crush it. The soldier was no less animated, picked up the tip of his nose and tossed it into the shop of my colleague, Mr. Galin, to run after his enemy. . . . When the soldier came to be bandaged, some wine was heated for his wound and his face that were covered in blood; then the tip of the nose was put into the wine to heat it up a bit. As soon as this wound was cleaned, Mr. Galin adjusted the tip of the nose to its natural place and kept it there by means of an adhesive bandage and a sling of cloth. From the very next day, the reunion seemed to take hold, and on the forth day, I thought so myself when I passed by Mr. Galin's and saw that the tip of the nose had perfectly taken and scarred.[28]

This relatively simple restoration technique marks the transition from the phantasm of a surgery of borrowing—phantasmagoric to the extent that the nose graft with donor represented the ultimate denaturation of Tagliacozzi's art—to the dream of recuperative surgery, a dream in which patients' intense desire to recuperate their noses is satisfied. Between this dream and that phantasm there is not the least space for the repair technique perfected by Tagliacozzi. The replanting of a separated nose depends on a practice employed by healers [*rebouteux*] because it consists in replacing a nose in its place by rebutment [*reboutement*], that is, side by side [*bout à bout*]. The ease, speed and effectiveness of this therapeutic act allow the nose to be repositioned. Confronted by a surgery that aims at revivification by reimplantation, Tagliacozzi's procedure is left out of the great art of surgery. It is an expression of the high baroque style in medicine, provided we keep in mind that this "handiwork" is perceived at the time, not unambiguously, as the expression of a virtuosity as unattainable as it is useless: "The Talcotian art does not, however, appear to have long outlived its author in Italy; nor need this seem wonderful, if we consider the extreme difficulty of executing it, and the very small advantages which it actually procured."[29]

In the eighteenth century, the art of surgery also relies on the theory of adhesive inflammation. One of the points under discussion is the treatment of cuts. In order to proceed to the union of the separated parts, the edges have to be brought together. Then nature has to be left alone to unite them through its own adhesive process. Once the nourishing juices provided by the blood have begun to flow, there has to be either a production of new blood vessels or an anastomosis with the old blood vessels. Hunter speaks of plastic, coagulable or organizable lymph. For Edward Alanson, one the most famous theoreticians of wound scarring, everything goes well and quickly:

> I have experienced the propriety of this treatment after lithotomy, castra-
> tion, the operation on the bubonocele, and many other important surgical
> operations; and have consequently procured a considerable degree of union
> by the first intention; a salutary result from the application of our dressings
> externally to the wounded surface; so powerful is nature in restoring recently
> divided parts, when not interrupted by art.[30]

This new way of treating wounds is so simple that it coincides with the kind of first aid anyone can provide—spontaneously. Heister reports one such case: "For I know an Instance of a Butcher's Finger that was cut quite off obliquely, but being immediately fixed, and retained in its proper Place by Deligation with a Linen-rag, it adhered, and became well without any other Medicines."[31] In 1759 Fleurant observes a case similar to the one Heister mentions. Pouteau has published his account:

> When I arrived, I found the patient's finger cut and, thanks to his wife's care,
> wrapped in compresses moistened with warm wine. . . . A quarter of an hour
> had passed from the time of the accident to that of my arrival. The fingertip
> was kept in place with a few stitches and, above it, I applied . . . compresses
> and a suitable bandage. . . . When after eight days I took off the first dress-
> ing of the wound, I found the parts reunited solidly enough to no longer fear
> their separation.[32]

Pouteau, it seems, is one of the rare physicians to establish a link between animal grafts and a surgery of replanting, even surgery with skin flaps that can be folded back if the cut-off part allows for it. He activates, in unison, a principle of conservation and a principle of exclusion. Pouteau associates vegetative life with the principle of conservation. The separated spur preserves a vitality that allows it to join again in the exchange of life with the comb. In the same way, any portion of a limb separated whole or in part, thanks to this vegetative life, is capable of uniting with the part that corresponds to it. The principle of exclusion concerns sensitive life. Animal grafts on warm-blooded animals take place without the participation of nerves: the engrafted part remains deprived of sensation and movement. In the same way, in the reattachment of a finger to the hand or of a tip to the remainder of the nose, it has been observed that these parts lose those very faculties. But we must not think that any cut-off part whatsoever can be reunited to what remains of the limb. It will never be possible to keep a cut-off hand or leg by sewing or bandaging it back on. And even if the limb took on, it would lack sensation and movement, it would not be good for anything. For a part to hold, it must be a small piece of flesh: the tip of a finger or a nose. In this requirement, Pouteau sees the providence of nature at work, a principle of compensation that, incidentally, also demonstrates the importance of the nose:

> All appearances suggest that the larger the portion taken off, the more difficult is the retaking. But it is easy to be comforted about the too narrow bounds of this vitality, which only preserves itself advantageously in very small portions. The deficiency in movement and sensation in the part that has been reunited with the greatest success would render it very cumbersome and completely useless, especially when it cannot have, like the tip of the nose, the advantage of obviating a deformity.[33]

If a finger that has been completely sliced off retakes when it is held in place, so must, *a forteriori*, a finger or a nose that is still attached, provided the wound is recent. It suffices to replace it and sew it back on. This operation consists in mending. To mend a nose is to sew it back on when it still hangs by a flap of skin. Loubet reports the case of a soldier whose nose had been detached by a halberd's blow: "I washed this nose, which was almost frozen and very cold, and little by little reanimated it with slightly warmed wine, and then made three stitches with an appropriate needle . . . I was extremely surprised to find the nose reunited and healed without any other aid, so much so it would have been possible to overlook the cut."[34] This account by the surgeon Hugues Ravaton is one among others:

> An officer of the Beuzenvald regiment in Switzerland gave the cook of the Commandant of Landau, who had undoubtedly been insubordinate at a village festival, a blow of his sword that cut off his nose. . . . The nose was attached only by a part of the right ala's skin. This nose was violet, swollen, and filled with blood. . . . I adjusted those parts of the bone that were pushed in, and adjusted the nose in its natural situation. . . . The wound had reunited and scarred well, without accidents or great deformity. . . . I have since reunited more or less similar wounds with the same method.[35]

At the end of the eighteenth century, Claude Antoine Lombard could write the following without running the risk of being taken for a charlatan:

> Many examples attest every day to the fact that, in order to obtain a scarification as complete as it is satisfactory, it has always been sufficient to bring together and carefully keep in place, with adhesive bandages and a well-thought-out apparatus, the lips or flaps of sizable wounds inflicted on the organ of olfaction. Even the cartilage, which gives so varied forms to the nose, has been known to be cut, torn apart and torn off without all hope being lost for the restoration of its primitive conformation. The lips of the wound properly arranged, the care of the learned and diligent man of art in a way perfects the work of their consolidation that is entrusted to nature.[36]

The surgical act of gluing a nose back no doubt has nothing extraordinary about it, provided we specify that it concerns wounds that are still open. To those who apply this readjustment technique, time appears as a decisive factor. Quick action has to be taken for the part to be replaced not to lose either its vitality or its warmth. The surgery, so to speak, has to take place while it's still hot. Cures, first and foremost, are immediate cures that are both simple and popular. Tagliacozzi's procedure does not fit this schema because it is free from its primary demand, urgency. But it is subject to a series of much more constraining conditions. Not only does Tagliacozzi's art call for highly developed skills, it is also destined for the aristocracy. Woodcuts show the different stages of the procedure, of course, but they also show the status of patients in a position to benefit from it: the residence is magnificent, the furniture refined, the clothing elegant. It is useless to insist on this point: the repair of the nose with arm flaps and the surgery of open wounds do not share the same spirit and do not apply to the same people.

The blindness toward the arm flap technique is quite understandable. Its motives lie at the same time in the fantastic, in empiricism, and in rationality. Tagliacozzi's art, altered by being associated with nose grafts with donor, topples over into a medicine of sympathies. Through its links with the marvelous, the procedure produces more and more disbelievers. In the *salons* of high society, the procedure is the object of ridicule. That is not all: animal grafts and the theory of adhesive inflammation highlight the theme of the repair of injuries without delay and through natural union. Hence the prevalence of replantation, the surgical act that becomes the procedure of choice. In comparison, the arm flap method appears as a curiosity. The use of repairing a loss of substance such a long time after the mutilation, and at so high a price, is not apparent. Does surgery that is more concerned with eradicating the signs of a deformity than with healing an injury still deserve its name? In the middle of the eighteenth century, Heister was unclear on this question:

> We have not yet acquainted you with the Method of cutting out a new
> Nose from some fleshy Part of the Body, and of conjoining it on the Face
> instead of the true Nose, which was cut or tore off. *Taliacotius* has a professed
> Treatise on the Subject . . . ; yet what is there proposed by the author, is, for
> want of later Experiments and Observations, judged to be impracticable, and
> without Foundation, by our modern Surgeons. When this member is lost, we
> must supply its Defect with an artificial Nose of Wood or Silver, unless, by
> being on the Spot, you can instantly replace and conjoin the real Nose just
> separated, either by Suture or Plasters.[37]

An infinitive epistemology in line with the philosophy of Emmanuel Fournier makes it possible to take the measure of such divergences and uncertainties. On the one hand, to repair, reform, restore, make, fabricate; on the other, to unite, reunite, join, readjust, rebut, replant, not forgetting, finally, to feign, simulate, mask, trick.

One may mock the metaphysical pose of a van Helmont who reflects on the destiny of a transplanted nose. To be sure, one must not confuse the notions of sympathy and antipathy with notions of immune compatibility or incompatibility. Certainly van Helmont's story of an allograft of the nose is a tale. But tales express a thinking of the possible. As for Butler, or for Voltaire who plagiarizes him, one cannot help but think of the deceiver deceived. In his *Handbuch der Physiologie der Menschen* [*Manual of Human Physiology*], Johannes Müller cites a remarkable fact pointed out by Franz Bürger. In 1823 Bürger announces the retaking of a nose that has been made from a skin flap detached completely, if not from the gluteus, at least from the thigh. But there's more: throughout the Enlightenment, recuperative surgery dominates the stage. One is tempted to say it constitutes the zero degree of reconstructive surgery since it limits itself to the application of sutures and adhesive bandages. Why try to force nature if one can just let her do her work? Why wait and end up applying Tagliacozzi's procedure when one can watch subjects recuperate their noses *completely naturally*? As long, that is, as one acts quickly, of course. What is at stake here, in fact, is nothing less than an opposition so paradoxical it becomes unthinkable: not an antagonism between a medicine of expectations and a medicine of actions but the exclusion of a surgical activism that has had its time by a recuperative surgery founded on a hurried naturism.

If we suppose that the past of a therapeutic practice blends in with its origin, we will see that this remote past and the actual present rest on the same *principle of indiscipline*. The development of the first notions of reconstructive surgery cannot be separated from a recusation of physical punishment as a shameful form of punishment. In the eyes of today's ethics professors, whose committees resemble tribunals, the realization of the first partial allograft of a face must contravene their prescriptions. If now we suppose that the history of facial surgery blends in with its beginnings, we will see that this recent past and our actual present have one thing in common—the idea of a partial allograft. We can leave aside the simple, elegant technique of the forehead flap: its reliability taken into account, this method of nasal reconstruction by autograft is imperfectible. In turn, it would not be wrong to suggest Tagliacozzi's procedure as starting point for a history of the face transplant. The Bologna physician is the first to evoke the possibility of a partial allograft of the face. Does he not claim to have refrained from performing the graft of an arm flap from a donor for reasons of simple convenience? Tagliacozzi's work, surely, belongs to the past of today's science.

THREE

The Face Transplant

At a conference in January 2006, Joseph Murray, Nobel Prize recipient for the first organ transplant (of a kidney between identical twins), reflected on surgical research: "Philosophically, once a surgeon has reflected on all surgical, ethical and moral aspects and arrived at a decision, it is counter-productive to second-guess. In fact, indecision can be destructive." So far, Dr. Murray said, the French team had "achieved a superb reconstructive surgical result."[1] The interview is still relevant.

The events are well known. A world premiere takes place on November 27, 2005: the partial transplant of a face (of the triangle chin–lips–nose) onto a woman with a serious injury. It has been foreseeable that this operation will provoke violent criticism from ethicists. They mount a full-on attack: The surgeons who perform this transplant are ignorant of the true medical problems, their behavior is unethical, and their goal is to achieve media success. In the eyes of those who present themselves as the guarantors of knowledge, morality, and proper publicizing, this premiere is disturbing. But it would be wrong to underestimate the force of their arguments. Their criticism is made with such clarity that it is possible to discern three series of questions they would like to raise in the debate.

The first set of questions is medical. They concern all the dangers the partial face graft entails. When an injury of the face is diagnosed, are physicians to opt for traditional solutions or to take the risk of going ahead with surgery? Is the procedure to be considered a clinical trial or a therapeutic act? There is a second series of questions. It concerns medical ethics. Do physicians, before they operate, have to be certain that the advantages of surgery outweigh its disadvantages or do they, on the contrary, have to take risks? Is a face transplant to be undertaken despite the severity of the required postsurgical treatment? The third series of questions arises from the relationship between physicians and the media. Are physicians to compromise with the yellow press and publish images of the procedure or are they to reject all publicity? Are they to communicate the stakes of transplantation medicine? All these questions deserve to be examined.

Medicine

The question of therapeutics is central. But everything plays out as if there was but one choice: either apply the habitual methods, without danger for the patient, or attempt a partial transplant of the face. In this schema, responsible behavior that respects the patient is the opposite of a medical activism in search of heroic deeds. To cast doubt on the expediency of a face transplant, it is necessary to believe that its purpose is to allay an inconvenience. Not only this, it is also necessary to think of transplantation as a technique with only one goal: to save a patient's life. It is necessary to believe that it is always possible to come to terms with handicaps as if, among these, there were none that are truly severe.

A short historical reminder is in order to better understand this attitude. In France, Article 2 of the 1976 Caillavet Law—later abrogated, then taken up again and modified by the 2004 bioethics law—states that "an organ to be used for therapeutic or scientific purposes may be removed from the cadaver of a person."[2] Leaving open the question of finality—"therapeutic purposes"—this article does not limit the list of organs eligible for removal. Twelve years later, in 1988, the most important interrogations concern scientific purposes, whose unpredictability is emphasized: "There is a difference between an organ *transplant* which can save a human life in the immediate future, and experiments for which the benefits are not predictable."[3] Here lies the source of all sorts of misunderstandings. The initial law text does not predetermine the goals for which one could proceed to the removal of organs. In the original *des fins thérapeutiques*, therapeutic purposes, the indefinite article *des* is partitive, that is, it allows for the application of the noun to more than one set of purposes. And yet a restrictive interpretation quickly imposes itself, as if it were a matter of course that only vital organs are transplanted. Imagination does the rest—hence the clear-cut distinction between the vital, the profound, and the hidden on the one hand, and the superfluous, the secondary, and the accessory on the other; between the grave, noble, useful surgery on internal organs and the superficial surgery on surfaces.

It is not surprising that medical conservatism has placed excessive confidence in traditional methods. Truth be told, the desire to stick with classical solutions like prostheses reveals a profound incomprehension. By associating a handicap with injuries that are incommensurable with damages to vital organs, one ends up no longer seeing the mutilation. Some are astonished that the patient has not been treated according to traditional procedures, as if this handicap were an injury that could be mechanically repaired. They do not see why time is a determining factor. In the eyes of the transplant surgeon, too many delays end up blocking the procedure. Experienced practitioners are well aware of the medical problem that confronts them. They know that time works against them: "The indication in this case, a recent bite not yet completely scarified, inscribes itself in a context of urgency: the more the patient's scarring advances, the more difficult the graft becomes."[4]

The conditions that allow for the realization of the project are far from indifferent for the outcome. For the theoreticians on the French National Consultative Ethics Committee, thinking consists in weighing. From the start, the ethicists' concern inscribes itself on the register of moral reflection: "Our pursuit is strictly of an ethical nature, i.e. [to] provide elements of [an] evaluation regarding the various components of the problem [that] would seem to us to have ethical value, and to weigh them against each other."[5] The verb *pondérer* used in the original report comes from the Latin *ponderare* and means *to balance* as well as *to weigh*. To describe deliberations that could precede actions as a weighing, a search for an equilibrium, is to privilege a situation of pure indifference amidst a universe without qualities. The idea of a perfectly indifferent equilibrium, as Leibniz tells us, is a fiction. This holds all the more for the idea of evaluating a fictive situation. And is this not, on top of that, a dangerous fiction? Does taking the time to deliberate on a scenario [*cas de figure*]—not on a defacement [*défiguration*]—not amount to a denial of assistance to a person in danger?[6] The lever, the practitioners' tool that serves to lift up mountains, is something completely different. The true relation of thought to action is of the order of judgment, not of deliberation.

To be sure, the conditions of possibility of the medical act are many, demanding, and delicate, a *complex* of thoughts that blends considerations of feasibility, preparation, time, and decision. These conditions are also philosophical. The task is to draw, from out of its own depths, the concept and value of the motive of a future act: to elaborate the representation of a face redone as best is possible. To aim for [*viser*] the restoration of a face [*visage*] is to consider a transplant to be *conceivable* [*envisageable*]. But without presuming a happy outcome (all the while knowing that the outcome may be tragic), without endowing an action with therapeutic meaning and thereby finalizing it, not all forces will be applied: for the outcome to correspond to the expectations, it simply is not enough to act with premeditation. In the case at hand, the outcome is uncertain. This leads to a dilemma: accumulate certainties or take risks? Display circumspection or audacity? It is easy to see on which side adventure lies. This does not exclude an acute awareness, on the part of those who fully live it, of the difficulties they confront.

The power of the refusal to take the smallest risk leads to a radical refusal to acknowledge setbacks, even to acknowledge human fallibility. Such prudence leads to a refusal of the very conditions of knowledge, conditions that sometimes are also conditions of therapeutic innovation. It would be naive to conceive of a way to align a surgical premiere with a procedure whose evaluation would show its benefits to outweigh its risks. How could anyone end up drawing arguments against the face transplant from an absence of

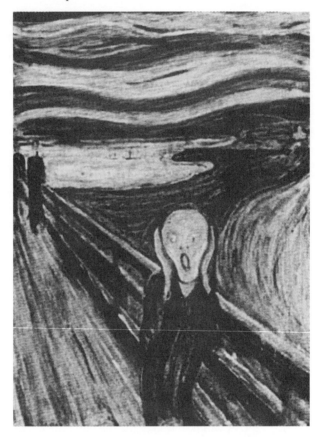

FIGURE 3-1. Edvard Munch, *The Scream*, 1893–1910, 91 cm × 73.5 cm (36 in × 28.9 in), National Gallery, Oslo. (Courtesy of National Gallery, Oslo.)

proofs of its efficacy, an absence proven by a lack of experience? If there is no experimentation, experiences will always be lacking. Whether we like it or not, to attain security, it is always necessary to first take risks. Uncertainty is at the heart of the therapeutic project. Canguilhem said that healing always consists in a decision to undertake, most often in an emergency, some kind of experiment for the benefit of life.[7]

The rift that separates ethicists and practitioners should now be obvious. They are completely opposed to one another on the subject both of the nature of the handicap and of the nature of the procedure itself. For the ethicists, what is inacceptable has to do with the conviction that transplantation is to be reserved for repairing the damage done to a vital organ that must at all costs be replaced. Conversely, what is acceptable has to do with the idea that the disfigurement is a disturbance that diminishes outward appearance alone, as if it were possible to believe that living with a severely disabling injury is simply living with a weakness of no great consequence. It is true, of course, that the act that saves is an act that ensures the proper functioning of the vital organs. Of course a heart transplant saves a life. But the living being is a whole. It would be absurd to separate organic life from functions of relation and to reserve transplants for those organs that are indispensible to organic life. We live thanks to our heart. But we also live on the limits of our body. When these limits are torn, breached, broken down, the unbearable becomes the unacceptable. But what is a life of relation for a disfigured living being? If, in René Leriche's words, "health is life in the absolute silence of the organs,"[8] we may say that in seeing Isabelle D., Bernard Devauchelle heard Edvard Munch's *Scream*.

Besides, it is no longer possible to maintain that the conventional methods exist to improve patients' quality of life. The value of a quality of life lies, above all, *in the living*. The question of biological norms might very well exceed the competence of those who present themselves as experts on norms. The disabled must be granted the right to themselves normalize their lives in relation to their individual potentials. To regain a face, is that not a way of normalizing one's life, despite all the constraints it implies? But who, then, is the most apt at evaluating the significance of a disturbance or the damage done by an injury, if not patients themselves? They can tell, without talking, where functional embarrassments end and true disability begins. Providing a solution for the disability that consists in a severe disfigurement is another way of saving a life.

It is difficult to evaluate the risks run by a patient in a surgical premiere. But that is no reason to rank such a premiere in the category of clinical trials. This procedure has nothing to do with a therapeutic trial for the purpose of evaluating a treatment. It has nothing to do with verifying the efficacy of a new therapy. Of course things become complicated the moment there is no statistical comprehension of an event. But it is not enough that a therapeutic act be without precedent for it to become a risky clinical trial. The partial face transplant belongs to the experience of reconstructive surgery.

A surgical premiere also is an experiment. But this does nothing to diminish its status as a therapeutic act. Anyone who would want to reject this double lineage would have to say that there is a history of surgery that is a history of routine procedures despite the fact that these very procedures, when they are performed for the first time, pertain to a history of experimentation. Put differently, one and the same procedure would figure in a history of experimentation as an invention and, pedagogically, in a surgical manual. This absurdity contains another: Surgery would have no history at all since all surgical premieres would slip through the cracks of a history of routine procedures. As for experimentation, its very reason to exist would become unintelligible. A surgical premiere constitutes at one and the same time an experimental and a therapeutic act.

In the situation discussed here, the task is to solve a medical problem or, if you prefer, to treat a severe trauma. The experts know better than anyone that no one experiments simply for the pleasure of experimentation. When professional ethicists exclaim, "That's experimentation pure and simple!," the aim is certainly to remind us of something so evident we tend to forget it, something physicians have been familiar with for a long time: to heal is to experiment. The only question one might ask is whether this or that procedure is harmless, harmful, or beneficial. To try to decide this question before the surgery is performed still blocks all questions: the question of experimentation, the question of therapeutic indication, and the question of the urgency of action. For the moment there is therefore only one certainty, which Claude Bernard invites us to share: "All those who restrict themselves to speaking of experimentation from the fireside do nothing for science; rather they harm it."[9]

The reconstructive surgeon belongs to a family of anatomists who would freely compare their successes to the exploits of navigators who discover new lands. Just as bringing to light an anatomical structure that has not been seen before is, in Gaspard Bartholin's phrase, an *ocular invention*, so a procedure that produces a face is a *manual invention*. As a sophisticated and complex surgical strategy, the series of acts that consists in preparing a part of the face in order to recover the face designates a creation. This creation takes the concrete original form of a transplant of *a* face. The essential point is this: a procedure differs from a protocol like the realization differs from reading a surgical manual (or from the *a priori* description of the conditions of a procedure). But there's more, namely a minute detail that, in the *execution*, turns out to be essential: the improvisational element that makes the event one of a kind. In this respect, the comparison with musicians suggests itself: "First decipher, then render the score and sometimes, if the score lets the imagination run free, improvise—in any case add a personal touch to it."[10]

This procedure also allows us to throw a new light on a central question of medical philosophy, a question that research administrators, concerned as they are with immediate results, have a tendency to underestimate. Canguilhem always insisted on this point: a nontheoretical activity, one centered on pathology, clinical care, or therapy, can be the cause of the renewal of a scientific problem. It would certainly be useful to oppose to administrators' rationalism, if not an empiricism then at least a "factual surgery" (Bernard Devauchelle). Does not the face transplant generate the kind of postsurgical situation that is also characteristic of spontaneous experimentation? This postsurgical situation has already proven to be rich in lessons for the neurosciences. The observations made on the way in which the motor cortex reorganizes corroborate and enrich the results obtained in the observation of cases of amputated hands.

The first face transplant has two more positive effects. On the one hand, it bridges the gap between transplants of internal organs and transplants of visible organs. Transplants of internal organs appeared to be a necessity, precisely because these organs are vital. The relevance of face transplants, however, did not become clear because, in Paul Valéry's words, "nothing is deeper in man than the skin."[11] But now face transplants enter the field of therapeutic transplants. It is no longer possible to believe that transplantation has but one goal, to save a human life in the immediate future. It must be acknowledged that saving a life also consists in doing everything to avoid its sinking into oblivion. On the other hand, this surgical world premiere shows what distance separates, at times, human experimentation from animal experimentation. This distance is the guiding idea of the founder of human anatomy. Vesalius, already, brought out the biological fact of human beings' singularity by underlining that the human being is its own reference, its own measure and model. This methodological rule applies to the face transplant as well, provided the *specific* problems it raises are taken into account. From this point of view, a snout transplant is of no interest. It is not by chance, then, that the first face transplant took place in a hospital, not in a laboratory.

Ethics

"Medicine may claim that it was the first activity to acknowledge itself bound by the principle of precaution. What else, in fact, does the Hippocratic *primum non nocere* [*first, do no harm*] amount to?"[12] From the moment one sees in Hippocratism an instance of the medical caution that is articulated in the principle of precaution, anything goes. The case of the face transplant thus becomes an example of choice: for the partisans of a kind of tranquil naturalism, such an injury of the face does not merit surgery. But there's more: given the dangers it entails, immunosuppressive treatment is on the same level as an illness. It's no good to get rid off a minor inconvenience in favor of a chronic condition—hence the assertion that it would not be ethical to offer the patient the option of a transplant. To maintain this point of view, it is necessary to separate immunosuppressive treatment from the therapeutic act to which it pertains. It is necessary, in other words, to abstract from the situation as a whole. Yet within the framework of the comprehensive attention that must be paid the patient, postsurgical treatment is simply a necessity. The argument can be turned against the detractors of face transplants: it would *not* be ethical to abstain from the initial procedure under pretence that the treatment turned out to be a constraint in the long run. To invoke the severe impact of medication in order to dissuade surgeons from operating is to incite them to renounce the primary duty to assist persons in distress. The appreciation what the advantages and inconveniences of a lifelong course of treatment are is also a decision on the part of the patient—in agreement with the physician.

The ethicists' reservations find a correlate in their complete adherence to organ transplants that save lives in the immediate future. Any act that does not conform to this goal would thus have to be excluded from therapy. But why should transplant medicine have to align with *reanimation* practices? Whether we like it or not, such a limitation tends to enclose transplant medicine within a framework that is bursting apart as it is. The concept *life*, in this context, designates a life under the conditions of *sublife*. The dogma of respect for life has to be questioned, particularly where it relies on a principle of indifference toward the conditions of living beings' existence. Therapeutic obstinacy is the act of *denaturation par excellence*. It, too, saves a life in the immediate future, by pushing back the limits of death. Yet it is clear that the ethicists subordinate medical techniques to a metaphysics of life.

Practitioners, in turn, make these techniques serve a physics of life. The procedure of the face transplant aims at a process of *renaturation*. To do so, all available resources must be brought to bear. The wisely armed art of the surgeon uses, orients, and supports nature with a view to establishing the return of impaired forms and functions. It would not be wrong to say that in this context mechanism and vitalism appear to be complimentary, as long as we specify that in the association of surgery and biology time remains no less an essential factor. Theoreticians of the security-minded approach who insist on the time of deliberation do not see that by transforming a treatment plan into a clinical trial project they have determined everything in advance. Taking an ethical posture leads them to turn a blind eye to the requirements of the very thing they pretend to defend, the interest of the patient. Neglecting the time factor in the face transplant procedure leads to reproaching physicians for confusing urgency and precipitancy. In transplantation medicine, there are procedures that pertain to emergency medicine. By the by, if health is a value, then *all medicine is emergency medicine*.

As far as free, enlightened consent is concerned, the ethicists are suspicious. Has the recipient been warned of all of the procedures' risks? Have all safety measures been taken? Have all papers been signed and initialed? Reticent as to the very idea of the face transplant, they have trouble understanding that a patient can accept it. It is naive to believe that such a project could keep its promises with a single written consent in conformity with whatever law is applicable in that situation. Is it necessary to recall that the treatment plan derives all its strength from the collaboration of each and every one? In the eyes of those engaged in the enterprise, the formalization of an agreement is a ridiculous procedure. The way to boost this project and to give it meaning again is to show how things end up imposing themselves, over time, in the framework of a collective adventure that brings together the physician, the patient and the nursing staff. This project has to be one in which each participant brings all his or her skills to bear. Free, enlightened, authentic consent exists—it is a tacit agreement.

The question of experimentation that is connected to the procedure seems equally delicate. This is a good time to recall that several physicians, aware of the risks they are running, have tried to shed light on a number of problems by experimenting on themselves. It might be objected, perhaps, that although auto-experimentation is an exemplary case, it does not justify experimentation on others. But experiments on oneself and on others obey the same principle. On the one hand, one must be in agreement with oneself to become the object of an experiment or the subject of clinical observation. On the other, to consent is to agree with one's physician: it is to agree with the projected procedure. Furthermore, if the patient approves the healing project, she does so not only because she is well educated about the dangers of the procedure. In the present case, the patient consents because there are affective ties with the medical team. It is still unclear why a surgical world premiere would raise such protest. No one is obliged to commend the patient's courage and the physicians' dedication. But neither is anyone obliged to disparage the medical team by casting doubts on the conditions under which the procedure is undertaken. To do so is unsound.

This repressive attitude is all the more arrogant for its reliance on psychology. Nothing more is needed to denounce the medical team's insolence. How could they perform so arduous a procedure on so fragile a subject? On a subject so fragile, furthermore, that certain newspapers went so far as to speak of suicide, not only of a suicide of the recipient but of the donor as well. Yet even if the information were true, it would not amount to an objection or a counter-indication. On the contrary, the failed suicide of the recipient and the suicide of the donor triggered events that should have swept the ethicists' fears aside. What is unforeseeable here is the reversal of situations. Thanks to organ donation, the suicide of the donor becomes a death that is as useful as any death can be in the eyes of her family. As for the recipient, she lives her disfiguration as an obstacle that has to be overcome. A transplant that would give her a face once more would end her suffering.

No longer indifferent to the way she looks, she once more cares for herself. After all, to have a reason to appear is to have a reason to live—despite new constraints. The life of living beings most certainly is more inventive than the schemata in which some want to enclose it.

Because they stick to present (or past) legislation in matters of bioethics, the public censors end up propagating strange ideas. Because they ask if the patient was well informed, they end up suspecting the physicians: Not only are physicians unable to manage difficult situations, they also do not know where the line is drawn that separates a useful procedure from all the others. The same presupposition is at the source of these rumors and serves to legitimate a crusade for the sake of public welfare: medicine does not think. To be more precise: it is the prejudice that medicine thinks *badly*. But a university hospital is a place where several competences converge, competences capable of uniting for the sake of seeing a project through. It rarely happens that a hospital shelters the secret lab of some scientist who is in league with the devil.

The face transplant has been the occasion for a recurrent theme in the history of medicine to resurface: you start experimenting on convicts, you end up experimenting on the little guy in the hospital. The latest avatar of this worn-out theme is the charge that it is only the great psychological weakness of the patient that has made the face transplant experiment possible. Once is not always, the ethicists reassure us. The patient's state of psychological distress has not led the surgeons to see her as a subject of choice for a dangerous experiment. We must invert the order of factors and modify them: The procedure is technically possible and is undertaken because it imposes itself in the interest of the disfigured patient.

We also have to brush aside the absurd and dangerous argument according to which it is necessary to be mentally balanced to endure this surgical ordeal. It is absurd because self-control could manifest itself as indifference toward one's appearance. If disabled people could always normalize their lives by the sheer force of their spirit, they would not need transplants. It is dangerous because to regard strength of character as a criterion of the right to have surgery is to base access to medical care on a form of meritocracy. The question of the right to medical care must not depend on the wealth any more than on the merit of a person. An economy of medical assistance that takes subjects' psychological capacities into consideration amounts to a selection. It is reassuring that, for the moment, the ethics committees have not proven that suicide survivors, drug addicts, and the mentally ill do not merit being cared for like other patients.

Most often, the ethicists start from the principle that all clinical cases that can possibly occur will find a legal solution in the voluminous literature they have selected. But a collection of texts ranging from the 1947 Nuremberg code to the 2005 Universal Declaration on Bioethics and Human Rights will never constitute a guide for action. The ethicists' argumentation is a move to legitimize medical ethics as an academic specialty. But there's more: to invoke texts to regulate questions that pertain to clinical experimentation is to block invention. What would happen if every medical problem had to be enclosed in advance within the confines of cases already adjudicated? There would be no more problems to resolve and nothing more to think. From the ethicists' intractable perspective, preference is due to the mutations of thought. As if by premonition, Bernard Devauchelle indicated the scale of the future act as early as 2003:

> Is it necessary to justify surgical premieres not so much because they are carriers of hope that in some way push back the boundaries of possibility but because, provocative as they are, they will elicit a number of questions that will allow for so much more progress once they are resolved? This would amount to taking sides against the law, to extricate oneself from the law only because that is the best way to make the law evolve.[13]

Do the ethicists remember the parents who, in the name of the freedom of therapeutic choices, wanted their son to have palliative surgery on a cancerous jaw tumor, a procedure that would reduce their child's suffering? Faced with a refusal pronounced after a pluridisciplinary coordination meeting at the Antoine-Lacassagne cancer treatment center in Nice, the parents turned to the courts. In a ruling handed down Tuesday, November 29, 2004, "the President of the Paris Superior Court declared the parents' petition to be 'inadmissible,' claiming that the State cannot 'interfere with the relations between patients and practitioners or with the exercise of medicine.'"[14] If the judgment about a procedure's relevance has to be left to the competence of the physician alone, it is unclear why a local (or national) ethics committee would have a word to say on the matter. Was it ethical to take on the case of this child as a pretext for some kind of payback? Was it really necessary to hide obscure corporate interests behind the hypocritical mask of enlightened compassion?

The ethicists should understand that it is ill-advised to deny the parties most directly concerned the capacity to judge a situation whose stakes directly concern them. They should also understand that it is presumptuous of them to prescribe rules of conduct in such situations. There is, at bottom, something contemptuous about those who know better than others what is best for them and what they have to do. With Descartes, let us instead bet on generosity because generosity keeps us from despising others: "Those who have this understanding and this feeling about themselves are easily convinced that every other man can also have them about himself, because there is nothing therein that depends on others. That is why they never scorn anyone."[15]

The ethicists believe they are in a position to prescribe the rules of good medical conduct because thanks to the collaboration of specialists with different backgrounds (philosophy, law, psychology, sociology, anthropology), they have an overall perspective on the situation. Compared to this, a medical team cannot but be ignorant of the magnitude of the problems. But what such a team lacks in extension it makes up for in comprehension. Its subject is not really the *social human being*, nor the *juristic person*, nor the *human person* but the *patient*. In the eyes of the ethicists, the transformation of the patient into the subject of a procedure, into an object of clinical experimentation, curiously appears as a grave assessment error. *For them*, this reduction serves to justify a medical act to be renounced. They do not see that without this reduction, there would be no surgery. The patient *is a medical problem*. What needs to be done for the patient to regain a face? It is quite possible to characterize the surgical act as a *heroic* act in the sense in which one speaks of dangerous, energetic, violent remedies. Physicians and their patients expect the best to come out of this act. There is nothing more to be said.

To the extent that it probably needs to be seen in connection with a suicide attempt, the present case very well demonstrates the perverse effects of the current system. Are the physicians to keep the secret or to choose transparency? Either they publicize the medical history in its entirety (including the circumstances of the accident)—yet then they run the risk of having to put up with a refusal. To speak of the patient's fragility is to give information that can be turned into an argument for blocking the procedure. If one speaks of a patient's fragility, it may be said *a priori* that an unfavorable opinion can be expected from any given ethics committee. Or the physicians remain silent about the context of the accident in the interest of the patient, since the purpose of the projected procedure is to disembarrass her. Yet then they expose themselves to the suspicions of the ethics committees and risk to appear as profiting from the situation and contemptuous of the patient. Naturally, such suspicions pretend to overlook that the patient's psychological reconstruction is one of the team's priorities. *A posteriori*, this leads to a judgment on mere—and alleged—intent. And indeed, the following question has frequently been heard: "Was the patient in any position to face the procedure?"

The physicians' position is not simple. Either they are masters of their own decisions and do not have to give an account of their actions. Or they must give such an account, and they are no longer masters of their choices. Couldn't we say of medicine what Aristotle said of philosophy, namely that it "must not receive any orders"? If it were necessary at the inception of an action to have all the knowledge necessary for its success, nothing new would ever be undertaken. Audacity is nothing without the ability to come to terms with defeat. Also, for all the repetition of the maxim that human beings must not be treated as objects, the objective is lost from sight. For all the deliberation on the means, one ends up forgetting that the physician's aim is to cure the patient.

Media

Very quickly, photographs published in a mass-market magazine are perceived as shocking, scandalous even—indignation on the part of those who assure us that such prints have their place: in scientific journals, not in the yellow press. This is one way already of acknowledging their demonstrative value. But these images also have a "prophylactic" value. Indeed, they make it possible to put an end to the denegation of handicaps that take the form of

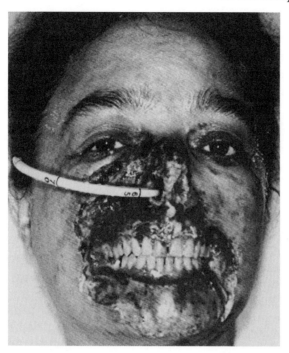

FIGURE 3-2. July 2005: Two months after being bitten by her dog, Isabelle D. lives at home and wears a mask when she leaves the house. (Photo courtesy of Service de Chirurgie maxillo-faciale, CHU Amiens.)

debilitating injuries. Before the surgery, viewing the mutilation interpellates the observer—brutally. After surgery, the face has a beauty close to that of the virtual and anonymous characters in digital 3D movies. The face is full, fair, and has a coppery tint. Its fine cut, like the stroke of a pen, traces the outlines of the parts, nose–mouth–chin. The necessity of the therapeutic act is no longer debatable.

These images indicate that the division needs to be not between an essential interior and the surface but between the normal and the pathological. It is also true that human beings marvel at their power to modify the face, to shape it like a work of art, to make it approach the form they aim to restore. Maybe we should say that the face transplant repairs and corrects at the same time. The value of health appears in its loss, the value of beauty in its lack. In the Renaissance, Girolamo Fabrizi d'Acquapendente said that true beauty and health stand in a reciprocal relation to one another. He added: "If this is true it would also be very true that the operations performed for the love of grace and beauty are also performed for the sake of health."[16] Inversely, as the face transplant demonstrates, there is no procedure of reconstructive surgery that does not in some way have to do with beauty. There seems to be a division between repairing a disfigured face and correcting some

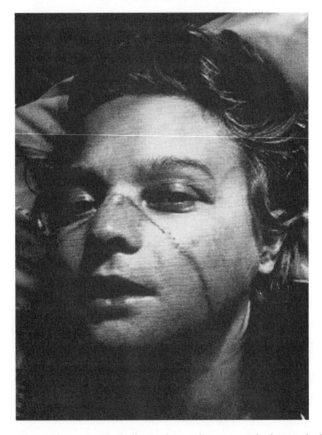

FIGURE 3-3. December 2005: Isabelle D. during her stay at the hospital, three weeks after the transplant on November 26. (Photo courtesy of Service de Chirurgie maxillo-faciale, CHU Amiens.)

imperfection. Yet the partial face graft is not indifferent to the harmony of forms. The relation between reconstructive and aesthetic surgery is not to be understood in terms of continuity. We can understand that the former includes the latter without, however, believing that the face has an aesthetic function.

For the photographs of the transplant to be even more persuasive, it is enough to show another set of images. Looking at some pictures of faces reconstructed with the help of facial prostheses, it quickly becomes clear that this surgical premiere constitutes considerable progress, perhaps even a gift medicine gives to her who no longer has a face. Surgery is an act of liberation. In Bernard Devauchelle's forceful terms, it allows us to be done with "natural straitjackets" as well as with the "anti-straitjacket." The term *natural straitjackets*, or imposed shapes, names faces both contorted by contracted, hardened muscles and put back into some sort of shape. The term *anti-straitjackets*, or masks, names "false faces" that liberate by imprisonment; they hide the disgrace. This, finally, is what makes this situation so delicate: the transition from the vital to the social. The skin guarantees bodily integrity. It is also the symbol of the human community and of its unity. Like the living body, the social body may be subject to fragmentation by breaks, rifts, rejections. To be without skin is to be skinned alive, it is a figure of social division and moral suffering. To be without a face is to be imprisoned in the very heart of the community. Michel Foucault would have said that to be without a face is to be a leper, dead to the community.

But it is not enough to show pictures to get rid of all the phantasms. Psychology does not lack the resources for inventing false problems and for unnecessarily complicating things. The following question has often been asked: "How can you live with a dead man's face?" We may rest assured: you cannot live with a dead man's face, because the dead have no face. It would not be wrong to say of the brain-dead human body what Aristotle said of the corpse: it is impossible to call it a human being other than by way of a homonymy, comparable as to its state of being, to a drawing of a human being. The body can of course be kept in a vegetative state. But it has lost that which made it a living body, an animated body. What is valid for the whole is valid for the parts, in this case a face that can no longer fulfill its functions.

The status of the graft is more problematic. On the one hand, if we look at its composition, it is a substance that lacks nothing. On the other, it must

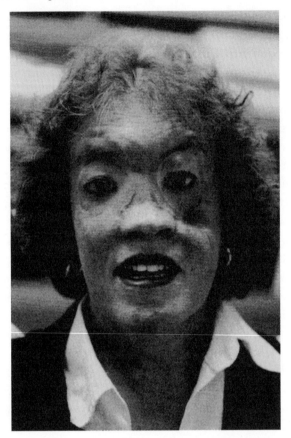

FIGURE 3-4. After being injured by a firearm, the patient lost her eyesight. Surgical reconstruction, then restitution with prosthesis. (Photo courtesy of Service de Chirurgie maxillo-faciale, CHU Amiens.)

be considered a living, albeit incomplete substance since it can return to the status of an organic part, a status it has lost at the moment of harvesting. Perhaps one should speak here of its vital power of reversibility, as long as it is taken care of for several hours. When the graft is harvested, everything changes. The same goes for the transplantation that restores its vascularization. Everything ends (or begins) the moment the surgeon loosens the clamps to restore its irrigation. Everything becomes animated. The transplantation triggers the graft's revitalization. It ends its hibernation. Then and only then is the graft no longer withered. Up until then, it resembled a mask cut from a rumpled rag. Very quickly, it develops, expands in all directions and obtains its final size, consistency and color, like Japanese dried flowers that unfold, swell, and take their final form when they are placed in water. Life "passes" from the donor to the recipient. Should we describe this moment in terms of appropriation? Nothing is less certain. We should rather annul subjects and "leave the infinitive with the possibility of being an impersonal without charging it with a heavily metaphysical and ethical meaning."[17] We should move toward a determination of being and think in terms of letting-be: *take off, put back on, transubstantiate*.

Certainly images often win out over an analysis of events. All they let come to the fore is emotive content. Close-ups shut out reflection. They fascinate because the face transplant connects with a dream of renascence, which is the negation of the limits life imposes on the living. It is a refusal

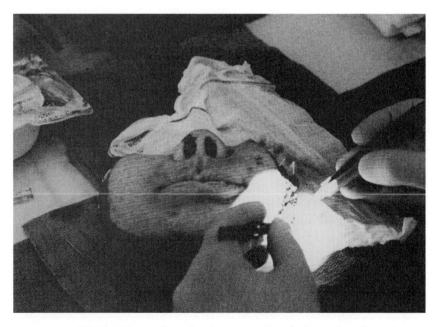

FIGURE 3-5. The facial transplant after harvest and just before revascularization. (Photo courtesy of Service de Chirurgie maxillo-faciale, CHU Amiens.)

of the disfigurement that presents the face of death, a death's head. It is as if one dressed in another's shed skin. It is as if one's shed skin becomes the lithe and silky garment of the other. Two myths collide. On the side of the donor a regeneration myth: for her family, she continues to live through the recipient. On the side of the recipient, too, a regeneration myth: the face of the other replaces the one that has been lost. Two destinies seem to merge and to blend.

But what is this procedure to be called? In France, the expression "facial transplant" [*greffe de la face*] has won out over very quickly over "face transplant" [*greffe de visage*] because phantasms had to be cut short. No one must be led to believe that the face could be interchangeable. Some base their choice on semantic motives, underlining that the word *face* is a scientific term that derives from classical Latin *facies*, which designates the "form or general aspect with which an organized being presents us." Others invoke highly metaphysical reasons. Sometimes they consider the face in relation to the exercise of an alleged physiognomic language. At other times, they underline

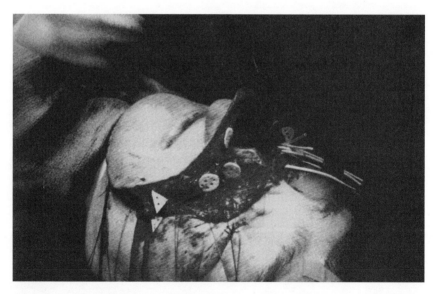

FIGURE 3-6. November 26, 2005, the moment of the transplant: view of Isabelle D. after the vascularization of the partial allograft of the face. (Photo courtesy of Service de Chirurgie maxillo-faciale, CHU Amiens.)

that the surgeon, who repairs the body, is nothing but a mechanic, and in this capacity he has no business dealing with the face [*visage*], which, as everyone knows, is divine. Everything that is essential has to do with speech.

These reasons are in no way convincing. First, a number of exceptions dismantle the certainties some have hoped to base on semantics. The word *face* appears with the meaning *visage*. It survives in this sense in the eloquence of the flesh to speak of God: The Holy Face of Jesus [*La Sainte Face*]. For Buffon, the word *face* has the meaning of *visage*: "When the soul is agitated, the human face [*la face humaine*] becomes a living picture, where the passions are expressed with as much delicacy as energy."[18] The adjective *facial* designates what belongs to the face. Émile Littré and Charles Robin refer to the article "Angle facial" [*facial angle*] for a "scientific" description that is not safe from theological contamination: The facial angle "very much approaches the right angle and is commonly around 80° in Europeans; it is no more than 70° in Negroes. It varies from 65° to 30° in the various species of monkeys and moves further and further away from the right angle as one descends the scale of beings."[19] Among the phenomenologists, we find the physiognomist Gaspard Lavater and the philosopher Emmanuel Levinas. For the first, pathognomy is the science of the signs of passions and of character expressions. For the second, the face is linked to humanity. His ethics privileges listening to the speech of the other: "This means concretely: the face [*le visage*] speaks to me and thereby invites me to a relation incommensurate with a power exercised, be it enjoyment or knowledge."[20]

The play of emotions, as a product of evolution, cannot be identified with the face [*face*]. Nor is it reducible to physiognomic language, and it has nothing to do with speech. In animals, capacities for facial expression are limited. But in humans, there is a genuine appropriation of muscular action for the purposes of expression. The eye is the "mirror of the soul" because the face receives and reflects the light of day and its shadows. Its modifications depend on the relief of its surroundings. The eye takes on the color of emotion as an effect of muscular actions. To ensure a major process of readaptation, one would speak of the necessity after a disfiguration to "envisage" a face transplant [*"envisager" une greffe de visage*]. The story can be told differently. The donor offers a face without eyes, a face flap. The recipient presents a lack. To take up the title of George Franju's 1960 film, she presents *Eyes Without a Face*. After the procedure, the recipient Isabelle D. recovers a face, a function of expression.

This facial transplant has brought back the question of identity. Several apprehensions have been voiced. The recipient might not recognize herself and might perceive her new face as that of another. One thing at least is certain: the recipient will not recognize herself as what she was before the procedure, that is to say, disfigured. But can the problem of identity be approached solely via the detour of one's self-image? Strictly speaking, there can only be identity in relation to images that serve as always-misleading points of reference. The living is never the same. Identity is the image the subject perceives as its appearance. Identity is also the representation of a being one wants to remember. In all cases, from the image of oneself to all forms of the representation of others, identity belongs to the imaginary. If we want to speak of what remains despite the wear and tear of the body, we will have no problem doing so once we dissociate the contents of our thoughts from the incarnation of our selves.

One could certainly also place identity on the side of the biological body. Identity would then designate what we share with others: the function of expression, this major adaptive process or innate baggage that gives us a selective advantage. The role of emotions could then be traced to two great functions, adaptation and communication. In the same vein as Guillaume Benjamin Duchenne de Boulogne, author of the 1862 book *The Mechanism of Human Facial Expression*, Paul Ekman retains six categories: happiness, surprise, fear, anger, disgust, and sadness. The contractions of designated muscles constitute units of action that express different emotions. What's more, this function cannot be distorted or obscured by social conventions. It constitutes a universal language.

Finally, one could place identity on the side of the textual body. A theory of appearances would account for this identity, an identity entirely relative since it is a fact of culture. It would be properly described as an identity by increasing individualization when it refers to the canons in effect in a given society at a given moment in history. Identity is accomplished in identification. The face, then, is the support, either definitive or temporary, of highly valorized signs, traces, or signifying marks. The spectrum is wide. It can reach from cosmetic surgery via different techniques of the body to Orlan's metamorphoses. In contrast, one could also speak of an identity by decreasing individualization, where the word *identity* designates the sign of what is perceived as the permanent identity of the subject. For any person, it is a fact to be a given individual that bears specific characteristics that allow the individual to be recognized by this or that agency. The spectrum is wide. It reaches from Alphonse Bertillon's forensic anthropometry to biometric passports via symbols sewn onto clothes, markings inscribed in the flesh and physical traits at one and the same time registered and constituted as signs of an identity.

But what drives a patient to want to recover a face? It is neither a loss of identity nor the wish to recover an image of the self. It could well be that what incites the patient is the desire to be done with the aversion towards oneself. The image reflected in the mirror triggers extreme pain. The image is shocking, unbearable. Dupuytren knew a lot about injuries to the face, the mutilations that give the face a hideous aspect: "These patients, who are objects of pity to all who see them, are an object of disgust and horror to themselves."[21]

As we come to an end, it is not without benefit to resituate this surgical premiere in its cultural, social, and political context. Kant had placed vaccination (which, too, is inspired by a gardening technique) in the rubric of heroic remedies. Canguilhem tells us that Kant attempted to define trials of new therapies on human beings, trials he identified as epic actions. Journalists were not wrong to speak of the first partial facial allotransplant as one that belongs in the category of heroic epics. It is, in all events, difficult to imagine a surgical premiere of this nature that does not lead to the patient's celebrity. Rather than attacking the perversity of the media, it would only have been fair to recognize that they did their job. It is to be hoped that next time, the public censors will show themselves to be more generous. This would allow them to avoid condemning the reading public under the pretext that they take pleasure from a medical adventure story.

Oh-so-virtuous souls were shocked by the fact that the recipient sold pictures of herself. There is a certain hypocrisy in screaming scandal when all this woman has done is negotiate with a mass-market weekly a deal involving a few photographs. Many who do not even need the money do the same thing. Another way of being outraged is to ratchet up the criticism and say that the face is not our property and that we share it with our fellow human beings. But we must not forget that men and women sell more than their image. Of course trading in our bodies or images does not prove that they belong to us; it only proves they have a commercial value for those who find themselves in a precarious financial situation. Of course selling our bodies or our images does not prove that we refuse to share them; it only proves that, in a social emergency, there is nothing to share. Let us also note, in passing, that bioethics is a luxury not everyone can afford.

The ethicists who have declared this surgical procedure to be a "spectacle" or a "media scoop" are completely right. We should recall that Galen, the most emblematic figure in the history of medicine, practiced in the squares and markets of Rome. It was there that he performed surgery, anatomical demonstrations and animal vivisections. Transplant surgeons follow their illustrious predecessor. The virtuosity of the surgical act is nothing less than an exhibition above which hover esthetic, affective, and cognitive values. But there's more: Galen sought the approval of his colleagues, of the elite, and of the people. Today, too, surgeons demonstrate that their therapeutic interventions are justified. It would be inappropriate to deny citizens the right to be informed or, in this case, the right to look. Why shouldn't the public be up to date on medical success stories? After all, there aren't that many. And then there is the fact that it is the public that finances the health system and, on occasion, some research programs.

This world premiere is one of those events that set in motion a discipline, its philosophy, and its image, all at the same time. On the medical level, it levels the chasm that existed between transplantations reserved for vital organs and surface surgery. Until now, the predominant opinion has been that repair by means of prostheses or autotransplants suffices for severe face injuries. Meanwhile, the jurisdiction of aesthetic surgery has been limited to faces in need of correction. The integration of a new reconstructive surgery into transplantation surgery not only signals a transformation, it also involves a new alliance of reconstructive surgery and aesthetic face surgery. The concepts *medication* and *medicalization*, too, reemerge in a new form: medication because immunosuppressive treatment is no longer seen as a danger but as a complement of the transplant; medicalization because the allotransplant is charged with resolving a series of problems such as troubled nutrition, elocution, and expressive functions.

From the philosophical point of view we must recognize that the trend of medical ethics signals an increase in negative, that is to say conservative, norms. In this respect, the surgical premiere has had the merit of shining a light on the "dogmatic slumber" of the ethics committees along with its correlate, a remarkable capacity for annoyance. At the other end of the spectrum, we find physicians for whom action is not a limited or delimited practice but a practice rooted in knowledge of the real and in the culture of the act. For them, it is not about multiplying obstacles or tracing insurmountable limits, but about opening up new problems and testing the possibilities of overcoming them. What Canguilhem wrote fifty years ago is still relevant to them: "Let's acknowledge the fact: In the text and in the prescriptions of rules meant to contain within the limits of moral conscience the therapeutic audacity so easily transformed into temerity by new medical and surgical techniques, there is today no qualification of competence."[22]

The publicity of the images is but a way of showing the necessity of the operation. They let us see how the choice to perform surgery could impose itself as the obvious choice on the surgeon. They also let us see that the face transplant is not about people who feel "uneasy in their own skin" but uneasy without their skin. These patients do not seek to improve their relations but to restore an interrupted relation. The sight of the photographs might offend certain sensitivities; that does not imply they ought to be censored. This procedure, like the publicity that surrounded it, resituates the medical question at the heart of public debate. It encourages organ donations. It desacralizes surgical practices. It brings an end to phantasms. It illustrates our modernity and establishes ties with beauty. What Baudelaire said of Constantin Guy in *The Painter of Modern Life* easily applies to Bernard Devauchelle: "This man . . . has a nobler aim than that of the pure idler, a more general aim, other than the fleeting pleasure of circumstance. He is looking for that indefinable something we may be allowed to call modernity." Things are born again on the face just as they "are born again on the paper, natural and more than natural, beautiful and more than beautiful, singular and endowed with an enthusiastic life, like the soul of their creator."[23]

The Manson Effect

The question in this chapter concerns the birth of medical entomology: How does Patrick Manson solve the major problem posed by the life cycle of *Filaria bancrofti*? He shows that the blood-borne embryos exit their host through the skin. The discovery of a new, airborne, and active host no doubt has a considerable impact on the history of parasitology. How does Finlay solve one of the great problems posed by the epidemiology of yellow fever? At the time, its mode of transmission is a true enigma. Finlay shows that mosquitoes lay several clutches of eggs and sting several times, and he dis-covers that their blood meal is linked to the propagation of the species; hence the hypothesis that the mosquito is the agent of the transmission of yellow fever. But it takes another twenty years before this hypothesis is verified by the Reed Commission and the life cycle of the nematode fully established. To be precise, it takes Ross's work on the life cycle of the malaria hematozoa to settle the question. Once the role of mosquitoes in the transmission of malaria has been demonstrated, it is possible to see the propagation of many other diseases from a new angle. Ross undertakes the conceptual conversion that Manson's method has made possible but not yet brought to light. Beginning with Ross, "the great induction," to use his own expression, names a structure of experience that will dominate exotic pathology. Research on filariasis fits into this structure.

An Epistemological Transformation

The events are known. In 1863, Demarquay observes worm-shaped creatures in the milky liquid he has extracted from a scrotum tumor. In Bahia in 1866, Wücherer examines the urine of a chyluria patient and notes the presence of small threadlike worms. In 1872, Lewis shows that these microscopic worms are to be found in the blood as well—hence the name *Filaria sanguinis hominis*. Shortly afterward, Lewis encounters these embryos in the blood and chylous urine of about twenty patients.

The parasite is known only in its embryonic state, until in Brisbane in 1876, Joseph Bancroft finds an adult worm in a lymphatic abscess of the arm. Shortly afterward, he finds four more in a hydrocele of the spermatic cord. He informs Cobbold of his discovery; Cobbold publishes it in 1877 and gives the name *Filaria bancrofti* to the parent of the embryonic forms, a worm thin as a hair and about four inches long. The following year, Lewis encounters the adult and sexed worm in a young Bengalese man on whom he has operated for elephantiasis of the scrotum. Manson confirms Bancroft's discovery. He finds parental forms of the little worm in different regions of his patients' bodies. All in all, as of 1877 researchers know that the embryos found in blood and urine are the offspring of an adult worm residing in the lymphatic vessels.

The discovery of the small nematodes finally sheds light on a series of pathological phenomena. Manson connects the disease called *Elephantiasis arabum* to *Wuchereria bancrofti*. He also considers hydroceles, cysts of the genital ducts, lymphatic varices and scrotal hypertrophy to be syndromes of one and the same pathogenic cause. The convoluted roundworms provoke a more or less complete obstruction of the lymphatic conduits and cause

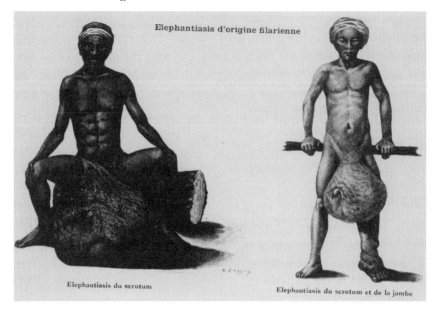

FIGURE 4-1. Filariasis due to Filaria *bancrofti*. Elephantiasis of filarial origin, elephantiasis of the scrotum (Victor-Pierre-Edmond Deschiens, *Atlas de parasitologie* [Paris, Deschiens, 1901], plate 31. Courtesy of Bibliothèque interuniversitaire de santé, Paris.)

inflammatory reactions that lead to the swelling and induration of the surrounding tissue. The deformities become permanent—elephantiasis of the scrotum.

Already in 1879, Manson is in a position to summarize the history of research on the filariasis parasite. Lewis has discovered the nematode's embryonic form and Joseph Bancroft its adult form. But Manson is the one who first describes the small worm's metamorphoses and establishes its life cycle. The development of the embryos cannot take place in a host who already harbors adult forms. The eggs of entozoa do not begin to develop until they have left the host inhabited by their parents; by the same token, the embryos of the roundworm must escape. This conjecture is founded on an analogy, but it quickly becomes a solid hypothesis. Manson calculates that there may be up to two million embryos in the vessels of a dog hosting *Filaria immitis*. Supposing that the microscopic animals begin to develop here before they have reached even a hundredth of the size of an adult *Filaria*, their total weight would surpass that of the dog—an absurdity that implies another: "The death of the host would imply the death of the parasite before a second generation of filariæ could be born, and this of course entails the extermination of the species; for in such an arrangement reproduction would be equivalent to death of both parent and offspring, an anomaly impossible in nature."[1]

To continue their development and to ensure the propagation of the species, the embryos must leave their first host; hence the idea of a cycle whose first phase consists in the exit of the microfilariae. In general, the embryos of endoparasites are ejected in excretion. They continue their development either in the environment in which they have been deposited or in the body of an animal that has taken in food from this environment. For a short while, Manson thinks the roundworm embryos could have taken the path of liquid excrements because several observers have noted the presence of the microscopic animals in chylous urine. But this mode of expulsion would amount to a pathogenic phenomenon much too contingent on chance. A process that ensures the function of propagating the species cannot be left to the mercy of an accident. And there is another reason Manson brings an external influence into play: The embryos are not equipped for leaving the circulatory system. They are prisoners in their fine sheaths (which are closed at both ends), passive and carried by the blood. The idea of wise and provident nature leads Manson to look for an exit path different from the one taken by most endoparasites.

The alternative, then, is as follows: the microfilariae are extracted either in bulk or individually. The first case implies that the embryos be extracted together with human flesh. The case of *F. sanguinis hominis* would be like that of *Trichinella spiralis*. Yet countries where human flesh is devoured are rather uncommon. Manson discards the analogy that implies cannibalism; the embryos must be extracted individually. The embryos' stay in the blood meanwhile provides a hint. If the first phase of the parasite's history unfolds in this fluid, the next must take place in the body of an animal that extracts it from the blood, in the body of a hematophagous insect.

But what parasites are free at every age and hungry for blood? "The privilege will be confined to a very limited number of animals—the blood suckers. This includes the fleas, lice, bugs, leeches, mosquitoes, and sand-flies."[2]

The choice must fall on an insect that is both abundant and familiar in places where filariasis is rampant. The disease is confined to tropical and subtropical regions; the geographical distribution of the insect that extracts the parasite must correspond to the distribution of the disease and the insect must share the same habitat. Since they are cosmopolites, fleas, lice, bugs, leeches, and sand flies are thus excluded. What remains are the mosquitoes—more precisely, the species of mosquitoes to be found in warm and humid regions. Two species frequent just the places where numerous cases of filariasis are found. Manson chooses the most common one and declares that the area of distribution of elephantiasis corresponds to that of the species *Culex mosquito*. Where the disease rages, these insects abound.

As early as 1877, Manson knows he has chosen the right species. He exposes individuals whose blood is infested with embryos to the bites of the insect. In the mosquito's body, he finds four times more larvae than in the same quantity of blood extracted with a needle: "From this it would appear that the mosquito has the faculty of selecting the embryo filariæ; and in this strange circumstance we have an additional reason for concluding that this insect is the natural nurse of the parasite."[3] In 1879, Manson establishes that the microfilariae have adapted to the nocturnal habits of the mosquito. The periodicity of the embryonic roundworm's life is a remarkable case of adaptation. At nightfall, the filariae begin to appear in increasing numbers in the peripheral circulation. Their quantity goes on increasing until about midnight (three hundred to six hundred parasites in a drop of blood). After midnight, the quantity begins to decrease and toward morning the filariae have disappeared from circulation for the entire day—hence the famous "law of periodicity," which confirms Manson in his choice of *C. mosquito* as intermediate host of the roundworm.

To follow the evolution of the embryo, it is enough to dissect the host at different periods of the larva's development. At the beginning of the first stage, the roundworm retains the form and movement it has within the human host. The enveloping sheath becomes more visible and an oral rim becomes discernible. One hour after ingestion, the worm sheds this sheath, and the buccal fold becomes more apparent. Then, very quickly, the larval stage begins. Manson perceives the isolation of the tail and the first traces of a mouth. The body shortens, thickens, and becomes transparent. Soon, the alimentary canal becomes visible. The last stage is character-ized by accelerated growth. At the end of the sixth day, the body reaches its maximal thickness. After a week, the embryo ingested by the mosquito attains maturity: "This formidable looking animal is undoubtedly the *F. san-guinis hominis* equipped for independent life and ready to quit its nurse the mosquito."[4]

But now a gap opens up in the life story of the parasite. How do the adult worms make it into the human lymphatic system? *In hindsight*, it is easy to see the answer prescribed by the logic of epidemiological perception. For those who practice this perception for the first time in the history of medicine, things are not as clear as all that. In Manson's view, the solution seems to impose itself. Since the mosquito dies just after laying its eggs, the filariae have to leave its corpse and thus have to be found in the water, there to lead an independent life. The rest follows: human beings are infected by swallowing water contaminated by the parasites. The invention of this mode of infection is founded on a three-fold perception. The first has to do with knowledge about the behavior of mosquitoes. The second depends on understanding the mosquito to be the nurse. The third is founded on an analogy with the life cycle of the Guinea worm, *Dracunculus medinensis*.

The first, disciplinary error is an expression of the times' entomological knowledge. It is thought that after its blood meal, the female mosquito re-treats to the vicinity of water to digest, lay her eggs, and die. Later, Manson deplores the absence of books that could have provided him with correct information, namely the knowledge that female mosquitoes can take several blood meals: "A regrettable mistake, the result of a want of books, was my belief that the mosquito died soon after laying her eggs." But Manson knows full well that it is not really necessary to justify his blunder: "For this error, I was not altogether to blame, for those books of natural history to which I had access gave little or no information about these insects, whilst one misled me by a very positive misstatement."[5] What Manson can have read is certainly not different from what Blanchard wrote in his 1890 *Treatise on Medical Zoology*:

> Two minutes are enough for the mosquito to gorge itself with blood.
> Weighted down with the weight of its distended abdomen and unable to
> sustain a prolonged flight, it will settle near stagnant water and rest as if

numbed: it digests the blood it has sucked and matures its eggs. After four to
five days, these operations are completed; it makes its way onto the water, on
the surface of which it lays its eggs; oviposition completed, it too falls into
the water and dies there.[6]

On the subject of the transmission of filariae, Manson is led naturally to
imagine a rather complicated procedure. To the mosquito as the first medium he cannot but add drinking water as the second medium. This joins
a whole new path of transmission, an active mosquito, and a classic path,
drinking water, because the female takes one blood meal, digests it, and dies
in the water, where she has laid her eggs. To account for this information
deficit, we must apply to the mosquito what Canguilhem says about the wild
animal: "For the human being, it is not only an outlaw of domestication, it is
a potential aggressor. Vital competition contravenes the contemplative attitude, the theoretical relation of the human being toward the animal."[7] We
find evidence of this attitude in Milne-Edwards's description of the behavior
of *Culex*:

> In the evening, they fly in numerous clusters and announce their approach by
> a sharp humming sound. Voraciously fond of blood, they pierce the skin with
> the bristle-like lancets in their trunk and distil venomous liquid into the little
> wound thus made, which causes vivid irritation and often considerable swell-
> ing. It has been observed that it is only the females that torment us this way.
> It is above all in the warmer countries, where they are called mosquitoes, that
> their attacks are to be feared.[8]

Claus takes up Milne-Edwards's description and in his 1884 *Traité de zoologie*
[*Treatise on Zoology*] goes so far as to say that the mosquito females constitute
"a veritable scourge."

At the time, it is unthinkable to endow these insects, which are already
perceived as harmful, with the even more calamitous role of propagator of
a scourge like elephantiasis. It is difficult to imagine that alliances between
living beings could to such an extent become disadvantageous for the human being. As we know, most often the identification of cases of adaptation aims at recording positive harmonies. Gardens, for example, appear to
be a peaceful and charming laboratory. The theory of pollination invented
by Sprengel is a model of explication based on recording cases of finality.

Underneath the bustling complexity of insects' collection of loot, Sprengel shows them also to be finalized for another activity. By transporting pollen, insects ensure the perpetuation of plant species. And as collectors of honey, are human beings not the ultimate beneficiary of this remarkable collaboration? Overestimating mutual advantages, humans are led to discard all thoughts of alliances detrimental to them.

It may well be that the principle of finality, which has shown itself to be so fruitful in explaining the exit of the embryos, ends up constituting an obstacle. Take this excerpt, in which Manson speaks of the adaptation of embryos to mosquitoes' nocturnal activity:

> It is marvellous how nature has adapted the habits of the filariae to those of the mosquito. The embryos are in the blood just at the time the mosquito selects for feeding. . . . When the mosquito penetrates a blood-vessel, the passing embryos, lashing about as is their habit, entangle themselves on the proboscis and get sucked up. Hence the enormous numbers of embryos in the mosquito's stomach and the selecting faculty of that insect.[9]

To account for the large number of larvae to be found in the insect's stomach, it is legitimate to evoke their behavior at the moment of the blood meal. There is no doubt the larvae have adapted to the insect's alimentary habits. But doesn't Manson go too far when he states that the mosquitoes are *finalized* to ensure the exit of the embryos? It is surprising to see him invoke a faculty of choice that allows the mosquito to select the microfilariae. Perhaps Manson, in his concern with explanation, overdoes it when he includes everything he sees in the framework of natural teleology.

The second blunder is complementary to the first. It is rooted in the belief that the filaria's metamorphosis is complete after one week. But it would be wrong to reproach Manson with bungling his observations or with lacking perspicacity, to accuse him of giving an incomplete description of the filaria's evolution in the body of the insect. The reason is that the lapse of time necessary for the larva's evolution has to correspond to the time that elapses between the blood meal and the death of the mosquito. This idea relies not only on a misconception of the mosquito's behavior. It essentially relies on the role Manson attributes to the insect, the role of a nurse. In the studies on the mode of contamination with filariasis this perception contains a conceptual blockage. All we have to do to discern it is to look back a bit.

In the Enlightenment, generation is identified with a kind of growth and fecundation with a kind of nutrition. The concept *metamorphosis* serves to designate the development of a preformed organism. The transition of the larva to the state of butterfly consists in shedding the wrappings that masked the presence of the butterfly in the larva. In the caterpillar, the naturalists already see the rudiments of wings, antennae, and legs. It appears in the form of a chrysalis, which is nothing but the butterfly still wrapped up—hence the term *pupa* from the Latin for *doll, little girl*. What's more, in the study of insect behavior, the raising of larvae by workers has led to these latter being named *nurses*. Réaumur writes about ants: "The mothers lay their eggs, . . . the hatching young become the great object of the solicitude of the workers, which are their nurses; and among insects and perhaps even among men it would be difficult to find any that are more attached to their nurslings and feel impelled to take such pains with them."[10] Bonnet for his part describes the different *modes of reproduction* of aphids: now by coupling, they are oviparous in winter; now without this help, they are viviparous in summer. Fecundation in winter makes it possible to make up for the lack of heat that, in warmer weather, ensures the hatching of the eggs in the mother's belly. But whatever the modalities of reproduction, aphids come from eggs: generation is identified with the progressive display of a preformation.

In the nineteenth century, *generation* no longer indicates the growth of a germ until it reaches the state of a new individual separated from its parent. The process that ensures the growth of a living being is distinct from the process that regulates the formation of the organism by means of generation and vegetation. In this new philosophy of living forms, the concept *metamorphosis* designates the life cycle of the larva, that is, an original individual's acquisition of form and structure in an evolution. From embryo to adult, individuality remains the same but it puts on different forms. In his 1842 *Om forplantning og udvikling gjennem vexlende generationsrækker* [English translation 1845, *On the Alternation of Generations*], Johannes Japetus Steenstrup shows that certain parasites give birth to beings that do not resemble their parents. The primitive type does not reappear until after a succession of asexual generations. He calls *nurse* (*nourrice* in French, *Amme* in German)

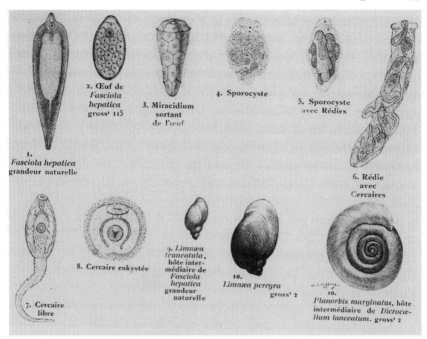

FIGURE 4-2. *Fasciola hepatica* and life cycle of the trematodes. (Victor-Pierre-Edmond Deschiens, *Atlas de parasitologie* [Paris, Deschiens, 1901], plate 21. Courtesy of Bibliothèque interuniversitaire de santé, Paris.)

that nonsexed individual that via the detour of gemmation gives birth to the sexed individual, and he calls *parent nurse* (*grande nourrice* in French, *Großamme* in German) the individual that gives birth to the nurse.

When Manson attributes the role of nurse to the mosquito, he uses a concept that designates now the workers of the anthill, now the sporocysts that live parasitically inside a mollusk. In the case of insects, the nurses' activity ensures the conservation of the species. In the case of the trematodes, the nurses guarantee different stages of the evolution of embryonic forms that lead back to that of the parent. From the egg to the adult form, the evolution cycle is complex. Miracidia, sporocysts, sporocysts with rediae, and rediae with cercariae are so many transitional forms that lead to metacercariae. Truth be told, it matters little whether the offspring that depends on the nurses lives outside the nurses as in the case of the ants or inside them as in the case of the cercariae that spring from sporocysts or rediae. What is essential is this: the nurses' activity is entirely provisional. The analogy between this biological phenomenon and a social practice (nursing children) contains another resemblance. Manson believes that the moment at which the filaria separates from the mosquito corresponds to the weaning off of the offspring. This idea weighs heavily in orienting his research. It certainly contributes to legitimizing the new question about the becoming of the adult worm: What happens between the moment at which the parasite leaves its nurse and the moment it invades the lymphatic vessels of a human being? "This hiatus is

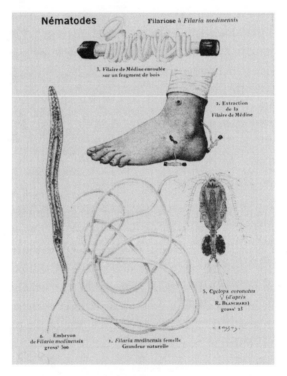

FIGURE 4-3. Filariasis due to *Filaria medinensis*. (Victor-Pierre-Edmond Deschiens, *Atlas de parasitologie* [Paris, Deschiens, 1901], plate 29. Courtesy of Bibliothèque interuniversitaire de santé, Paris.)

not likely to be filled in, except by conjecture, conjecture founded, however, on, and borne out by, analogy."[11]

The third blunder is all the more inevitable, since a parasite in the water evokes the idea of contamination by way of this medium. Chance is not involved. The very first discovery concerning the life cycle of filariae has just been made by the Russian naturalist Alexei Pavlovich Fedchenko. It has always been known that dracunculiasis is caused by the Guinea worm (*Dracunculus medinensis*). This parasite's life cycle presents a particularity: the female lives in the dermis and contains thousands of larvae that she liberates upon contact with water. Around 1870, Fedchenko's research turns to crustacea as possible intermediary hosts. The idea, based on a resemblance between the embryos of *Dracunculus medinensis* and those of the perch parasite *Cucullanus elegans*, has been suggested to him by Leuckart. The larvae of *Cucullanus elegans* emigrate into the body of a small crustacean of the genus *Cyclops*, in whose visceral cavity they undergo a double molt. Their definite organization, however, they acquire in the intestines of the perch that swallows the crustacean along with its cargo of larvae and thus infects its flesh with parasites. Cobbold emphasizes Leuckart's decisive role: "The Russian traveller was led up to his discovery by the previous investigations of Leuckart respecting the young of *Cucullanus*. The Leipsic helminthologist had, indeed, specially instructed Fedchenko as to the probable source of *Dracunculus*. It is often thus that science makes its clear advances, since a master-mind is needed to set others on the right track."[12]

It is only natural, then, for Manson to establish an analogy between the life cycles of *F. bancrofti* and *D. medinensis*. The latter completes its cycle in the *Cyclops*'s body, where it undergoes a metamorphosis, transitions to the larval state, and becomes a small nematode. Humans are infected by drinking water contaminated by the *Cyclops*. The larvae escape from the small crustacean during digestion and emigrate through the walls of the duodenum to then lodge themselves in the dermis. *F. bancrofti*'s cycle, unlike that of *D. medinensis*, does not require the ingestion of its nurse. In fact, *F. bancrofti* reaches the adult stage at the very moment its nurse dies in the water. The filaria devours the insect's tissue and begins an independent life in the water. It is probably by way of a detour through drinking water that it makes its way into its definitive host: "Escaping into the water in which the mosquito died, it is through the medium of this fluid brought into contact with the tissues of man, and then either piercing the integuments, or, what's more probable, being swallowed, [the filaria] works its way through the alimentary canal to its final resting place."[13]

It is easier to see now why the identification of the mosquito as a nurse brings with it both an unprecedented opening in the history of the formation of the concept of a vector and a spectacular conceptual blockage. It provides an opening because for the first time the mosquito is perceived as the organism inside which the evolution of filaria larvae takes place. There is no doubt that the relation between the insect and the nematode's larvae belongs to the domain of adaptation between two different zoological species. But this relation needs to be thought within the framework of a problematic of intermediate hosts. This point is not lost on Cobbold. At a time when Manson still speaks of *nurses*,[14] Cobbold substitutes the term *intermediary host*: "The character of the changes undergone by the microscopic *Filariæ*, and the ultimate form assumed by the larvæ whilst still within the body of the intermediate host (*Culex mosquito*), are amply sufficient to establish the genetic relationship as between the embryonal *Filaria sanguinis hominis*, the stomachal *Filariæ* of the mosquito, and the sexually mature *Filaria bancrofti*."[15]

By another detour, the perception of the mosquito as a nurse brings with it a conceptual blockage. The idea according to which the mosquito serves as a nurse turns out to be deleterious. The question is no longer *how* the threadworm closes its life cycle but *when* and *why* it must leave its nurse. Manson thus puts the answer into the question, and what he thinks of as a solid body of evidence testifies to this. He bases his conviction on the observation of a series of simultaneous events: the death of the mosquito, the adulthood of the threadworm, and its migration into the water. Twenty years later, Ross will brush all of this aside (which earns him the Nobel prize). But I don't want to get ahead of myself. Understanding that the worms do not leave the insect and that it is the insect that ejects them is no negligible task.

A Relocation

At first, medical science views the problem of the etiology of yellow fever from the angle of the theory of parasites. At the time, the pathogenic agent of yellow fever is supposed to be a specific germ, a hypothesis based on the observation of pathologic phenomena whose sequence and regularity speak to a specific cause. Two complementary reasons reinforce this etiology: on the one hand immunity, the fact that a single attack seems to protect individuals from a new infection; on the other the idea that the pathogenic agent must be mobile since it seems to attach itself to bodies and objects. Yellow fever thus enters the framework of parasitic diseases. The agent is specific, that is to say, it transmits yellow fever but no other disease. What's more, this cause multiplies as it spreads, which is a particularity of living organisms.

But the specificity of the cause is not a sufficient reason to identify yellow fever with an infectious disease. An affection can be declared contagious when the virus has entered a patient's body and symptoms appear promptly. Yet the physicians who are confronted with cases of yellow fever state that the individuals who are most exposed do not always contract the disease. They note that attempts at contamination by way of materials thought to carry the germ have failed. Furthermore, numerous observations show that a considerable amount of time can pass between the exposition of a ship in a port where the disease rages and the appearance of the disease on board. The yellow fever toxin, unlike the variola virus, must be developed and maintained outside the body.

Several significant data finally emerge from epidemiological studies. The scourge seems to depend on the insalubriousness of vessels and on a hot, humid climate. Hence the identification of the pathogenic germ with a vegetal organism: its mode of action is explained with the help of the history of inferior plants' generation. The germs could be brought, in a dormant state, onboard a ship and there, sooner or later, find conditions conducive to their reviviscence: "The poison manifests itself under certain conditions, such as are favorable to the growth of organic life, namely, a temperature above 72° Fah., moisture, and the presence of decomposing organic matter."[16]

But it quickly becomes clear that the factors usually invoked are not sufficient to reveal the infectious principle. On the one hand, insalubriousness does not always entail the appearance of the disease. During crossings to India or China, the worst sanitary conditions on board have never provoked the epidemic. On the other hand, many regions have climates that would favor the disease and yet are not affected by it. The majority of physicians perceives this strange characteristic of yellow fever. The consequence they quickly draw is this: if the disease does not show despite all favorable circumstances, the action of an additional factor must be presupposed.

The hypothesis according to which the germs acquire their virulence in the environment does not exclude a human filiation. It is possible, without contradicting oneself, to admit this extracorporeal transformation of the yellow fever germ and also to reactivate the idea that it comes from a patient. This, to be sure, posits an indirect filiation, since the transformative power of the environment has to be brought into play between the moment the germs detach from the patient and the moment they infect the healthy individual. For Bemiss, the toxin is reproduced inside the organism. After detaching itself from the diseased body, it must undergo a transformation that increases its harmful properties. The American physician aligns yellow fever with indirectly transmissible diseases: "Dr. Bemiss is one of the few observers of great experience and high authority who hold a contrary opinion. 'It [the toxin] is reproduced chiefly, if not wholly, within the body, but,' as he goes on to say, 'undergoes some change after its escape from the body, which increases its toxic qualities.'"[17]

Meanwhile Bemiss encounters the same difficulty as the proponents of the infection hypothesis. He fixes on the nature of the factor likely to determine the germ's virulence. Things are somewhat clearer when it comes to the mode of propagation. Like his colleagues, Bemiss speaks of the respiratory tract: "There is . . . abundant evidence that the disease is usually contracted by inhaling infected air. Yellow fever must be numbered among those epidemic maladies whose special poisons are air-borne, and through that medium distributed."[18] All in all, Bemiss's response is faithful to the theory of the *nidus*, a term that early on acquires the meaning, both figurative and abstract, of "an environment that is favorable to the eclosion of something." In medicine, Pettenkofer connects the nidus theory with the factor that triggers the germ's toxicity, a hypothesis supported by the Munich School. The German doctor seeks to account for the apparent yet inexplicable capriciousness of some of the great cholera epidemics that ravage Germany. There is no doubt that the germs of cholera reside in patients' excretions, but in order to become harmful, they need to undergo a maturation in the ground soil that endows them with their full virulence. In a next step, these germs, mixed with the emanations of the soil, rise into the atmosphere and penetrate human dwellings. The condition of the soil beneath sites and houses seems to play a determining role. What counts is not the soil's geological nature but its physical state. Chalky soil, hard rock, dried silt impart immunity. In turn, sandy or pebbly ground, porous, clayey, humid, and water-filled soils are dangerous. Cholera germs from excrement filter into these soils that are conducive to their maturation, which is why they are toxic, as Griesinger elaborates:

> What is harmful in all these cases is less the humidity of the air, which is greater in proximity to water, than the ground water . . . , which maintains a constant humidity in the foundations of houses, in cellars, and on the lower floors and which mightily boosts the putrefaction of organic materials in the soil.[19]

I will now return to how the hypothesis of the mosquito as agent of transmission is formed. To begin with, it presupposes a reflection on the problem of the extracorporeal transformation of the yellow fever germ. Finlay finds this question in the Plymouth Report, submitted to the US Department of the Navy in May 1880: "This [the discovery of the yellow fever mosquito] happened about the time when Bemiss, Stone and other American yellow-fever experts had invented the 'nidus theory' . . . I had, however, conceived a different solution of the problem. My own conclusion had been that . . . the natural transmitter of the disease must be a blood-sucking insect."[20] But when Finlay says he has come up with a different solution, he skips all the steps that make it possible to understand how he proceeds—four steps, to be precise. The first consists in showing that Bemiss's theory cannot apply to yellow fever. The second step is the substitution of Manson's theory for Bemiss's: a dead end. The third marks a change of direction. Finlay still applies Manson's theory but this time to solve the problem of the transmission of the disease: another dead end. Yellow fever cannot have water as its ultimate medium. What remains is the mosquito. Hence the fourth and last step that concludes with a success and with a defeat: a success because the mosquito is identified as the agent of the transmission of yellow fever; a defeat to the extent that Finley identifies the mosquito as a mechanic carrier. To understand Finlay's contribution to medical entomology, it is necessary to briefly revisit these four steps.

The nidus theory suggested by Bemiss is given as a solution for the problem of the extracorporeal transformation of the yellow fever germ. The corollary of this theory is a mode of transmission based on the inhalation of the pathological agent via the respiratory tract. Finlay considers this mode of propagation, which presupposes the diffusion of the germ in the atmosphere, to be improbable. He brings up a series of observations to counter Bemiss's theory. The atmosphere is not the vehicle of germs since ships that have no communication with the coast are not affected. Furthermore, winds do not influence the spread of the affection. The atmosphere is not the vehicle of the germs because there are no germs in the atmosphere. And neither is the nidus.

Finlay answers the question of the extracorporeal transformation of the germ with the theory Manson has elaborated to explain the life cycle of the threadworm. He identifies the mosquito with the nidus. The insect's body is the environment in which the germs seek shelter, settle, and reach maturity, which coincides with their dangerousness. But Finlay soon discards this new hypothesis because the yellow fever germ cannot be found in the blood of patients. This negative result blocks the answer to the question of the yellow fever germ's extracorporeal transformation. It would be absurd to maintain that the mosquito is the intermediary host of a pathogenic agent whose nature is unknown.

Finlay turns to the only problem that can be analyzed: the mode of yellow fever's propagation. To resolve it, he once again applies Manson's theory. The mosquito with its cargo of parasites comes to die on the water: the filaria escape and a human being swallows the water thus contaminated. To be sure, the yellow fever germ cannot be found; but one may admit, as a hypothesis, that the pathogenic agent is to be found in patients' blood. Hence the alignment of the mode of transmission of yellow fever and filariasis and the correlative duplication of Manson's theory in a Finlayean version. If yellow fever is transmitted via drinking water, then this water is contaminated either (if the mosquito dies quickly) by virulent blood it had extracted from a human or (if it survives) by excrement it ejects. Yet the Finlayean version of Manson's theory recalls the mode in which cholera is propagated. If the germ resides in the endothelium, which lines the walls of blood vessels, yellow fever can easily be aligned with cholera when it comes to the mode of transmission. Yet Finlay knows that the epidemiology of yellow fever contradicts the idea that it spreads like cholera, i.e. through the ingestion of water contaminated by excretions of those infected.

Once Finlay shows that yellow fever, unlike filariasis, does not ultimately pass through water, the mosquito as first medium is equally useless. But the mosquito does become necessary if yellow fever is brought upon a healthy individual after its first blood meal, which gives rise to the hypothesis of the *Culex* mosquito as the agent of transmission. Finlay comes up with the idea that viruses are transported from infected tissue (the vascular endothelium) into the corresponding tissue in a healthy individual. Finlay thinks of the old technique of inoculation in the form of a *natural* inoculation. This identification of the mosquito with a syringe once again provides an opening and puts up an obstacle. There is an opening to the extent that Finlay attributes a major role to the mosquito. For Manson, the mosquito has the status of a nurse and a first medium. Thanks to Finlay, the mosquito becomes the only medium. There is an obstacle because identifying mosquito and syringe leads Finlay to confuse an improbable vaccination with an experimental demonstration.

To get to the essential point: The mosquito serves as a vehicle if it multiplies its bites. This gives rise to the question why the female absorbs so much blood, which in turn provides a new framework for research: the information that could provide a basis for the hypothesis belongs to entomology. Finlay knows that a female captured in the act of fecundation and separated from the male takes several blood meals. So much blood cannot serve to feed so small a body:

> I have come to the conclusion that the sucking of blood is intended for another object connected with the propagation of the species. . . . If, for instance, the maturation of the ovules contained in the ovaries of the mosquito demands a temperature of 37° C., the latter could scarcely be obtained by any other means so readly [*sic*] as by the insect filling itself with a fair amount of blood of that temperature . . .
>
> Evidently, from the point of view which I am considering, the *Culex* mosquito is admirably adapted to convey from one person to another a disease which happens to be transmissible through the blood.[21]

Species of a larger size can absorb all the blood necessary for the maturation of all eggs in one single blood meal. They lay them all at once. Smaller species like the *Culex* mosquito, however, need to fill up several times and lay their eggs in several sessions.

Finlay shows that the geographic distribution of the disease can be superimposed on that of the mosquito. He notes that the seasons offer conditions that favor the insects' activity at some times and hinder it at others. Sometimes the epidemic abates in close proximity to its point of origin because the action radius of the insect is limited: the *Culex* mosquito is a bad glider. Furthermore, its females never stray far from water. This leads to the study of the topology of larvae's habitat. Finally, it may happen that the affection spreads to places far away from its point of origin. Hidden in a piece of clothing stored away in a trunk, mosquitoes could travel. This nesting of vehicles accounts for the irruption of yellow fever in European and American ports. Thanks to the attention he pays to the insect's many biological particularities, Finlay articulates notions that are indispensible for understanding the mosquito's intervention in the pathogenic complex.

To sum up: female mosquitoes suck blood to ensure the maturation of their eggs. The *Culex* mosquito especially takes several blood meals and lays eggs several times. On the one hand, the identification of the mosquito with a syringe allows Finlay to correct Manson's theory. On the other, this identification complicates everything. Finlay, incidentally, is well aware of the weak point of his hypothesis. If its sucker can serve as a syringe, the mosquito can transport any pathogenic germ whatsoever. What's more, any species of bloodsucking insect could spread the yellow fever agent. To sidestep these difficulties, Finlay is led to attribute a double function to the insect's salivary secretion: an elective function, in that it offers yellow fever germs a "germinative" property, and a selective function, in that it is a "bactericide" for all other germs.

It has gone unnoticed that the same year that Finlay publishes his hypothesis about the role of the mosquito, in 1881, Dimmock publishes his dissertation, *The Anatomy of the Mouth-Parts and of the Sucking Apparatus of Some Diptera*, which he writes under the direction of Leuckart and defends at Leipzig University. Howard, one of the most eminent authorities in matters of medical entomology, is known to have spoken of Dr. Dimmock's "admirable dissertation."[22] Dimmock's research undeniably stands in the tradition of the great entomologists Réaumur, Fabricius, Gleichen, and Meigen. He is the first, it seems, to provide experimental proof for a hypothesis formulated and discussed by his predecessors. The inflammation that follows a bite is not the result of mechanic irritation but depends on the secretion of a toxin. This toxin is discharged into the wound only during a blood meal, which gives rise to the idea that this irritating toxic substance serves to liquefy the large quantity of blood absorbed by the female mosquito. In the eighteenth century, Réaumur suggests as much to solve a problem linked to the absorption of blood:

> It is very apparent that our blood does not possess the degree of fluidity it needs to have to flow into the sucker of the gnat, which, before it attempts to introduce blood into the sucker, mixes the blood with a very liquid water. This water, furthermore, may be necessary to temper the blood on which the gnat feeds. . . . The gnat, which does not have any teeth and does not need any to work on the liquid food it passes into its stomach, imbibes this food, our blood, with a liquor fit to ferment it.[23]

Dimmock, for his part, multiplies the proofs. When a mosquito bites the skin without the sucker penetrating into a blood vessel, redness is slight and passes quickly. When it fills up with blood, on the contrary, the inflammation linked to the secretion of the toxin is obvious: "The above-mentioned facts would indicate a constant outpouring of some sort of poisonous fluid during the blood-sucking process, and would necessitate a tube or channel for its conduction."[24] But there's more: Dimmock confirms the idea that the female, unlike the male, feeds on blood. It is thus important to compare the buccal apparatuses of males and females. The males' apparatus is not equipped with mandibles that would allow it to penetrate the skin. A second, complementary observation concerns its behavior: the male is not attracted to human beings. If you place a glass filled with males open side down on the back of the hand, the males never bite. Dimmock is thus led "to suppose that they take a smaller quantity of food than the females do, and that they do not obtain it by piercing the skins of animals."[25]

Dimmock's work, to be sure, belongs to natural history, yet it leaves out one central question: Why do the females feed on blood? For Dimmock, blood intake *is food intake*. It could well be that the rather eloquent expression "blood meal" has contributed to confusion in the matter. Actually, it could not be otherwise. Dimmock's ingenious experiments are made within the framework of an exploration of the function of nutrition—to witness, the fact that he compared male and female under the triple aspect of buccal apparatus, the nature of the food, and the mode of food intake. It is clear that this comparative study of the nutritive function *from the first* bars the question why the female absorbs so much blood. As long as the answer is implied in the question, the digestive apparatus remains the only object of study. Paradoxically, Dimmock's work serves to reinforce a belief widespread among his contemporaries. Later, Howard describes the misconception: "There used to be a current idea that when a female mosquito sucks a full meal of blood she is never able to bite again, since it was thought that she is unable to digest such a meal. This idea, however, has been exploded in the experimental medical work."[26] Not only is it believed that the female dies after laying her eggs, she dies of indigestion!

Paradoxically it is because he focused his attention on an epidemiological problem that Finlay can conceive of the blood meal from the perspective of the function of propagation. But not until the turn of the century is his point conceded. Some succinct formulae deserve being cited: "Previously fed and fertilised insects would lay a second batch of eggs after a second meal of blood without a second fertilisation; but never laid a second batch of eggs without a second meal of blood. That is, one fertilisation suffices for several batches of eggs but one meal of blood for only one batch of eggs. . . . In other words *the insects need blood for the propagation of their species.*"[27]

The Great Induction

Twenty years pass before the Reed Commission, after and according to Ross, proves that the *Culex* mosquito is indeed the vector of yellow fever. Naturally, the same amount of time passes before the question of *F. bancrofti*'s life cycle is settled. To make the viscosity of time palpable, we need to show that work on the agent of malaria occupies a very important position in medical research. From 1880 to 1898—the names of Laveran and Ross can serve as reference points—research on malaria reveals its fecundity. Just as Manson's work makes it possible to understand how Finlay conducts his work, so Ross's work makes it possible to capture the work of the Reed Commission on yellow fever and Low's work on filariasis. What follows is a short description of the process that finally balances the perception of tropical medicine.

In 1880, Laveran discovers and describes the malaria parasite genus *Plasmodium*. These parasites live in the blood cells of infected patients. In the years that follow, Golgi brings order into Laveran's observations by arranging them in a cycle that traces the parasites' schizogony. This work leads to the articulation of some important laws concerning this group of organisms. But the work done by Laveran and his immediate successors leaves two problems unsolved. The first problem concerns the nature and role of certain forms of the parasite that eject long, mobile filaments. In blood drawn from patients, does one observe in these forms disintegrating bodies or rather a new stage in the development of the parasite? Grassi and Bignami believe they are dealing with a degeneration phenomenon. Laveran, Golgi, Danilewsky, and Pfeiffer think these bodies play a role in the transition from the parasite's corporeal to its extracorporeal stage. There is another question: how does the disease spread? Malaria infection has been successfully replicated by inoculating healthy individuals with the blood of malaria patients; apart from this artificial path of infection, the disease does not appear to be directly communicable. Do the parasites live as saprobes in stagnant water? Do they penetrate the organism by way of the ingestion of diseased water or by way of the inhalation of dust from dried-out swamps? Other paths are suspected as well. Bignami takes up King's old idea that the parasite infects mosquitoes that carry it from the swamps to the human being. Conversely, Laveran and Kock say mosquitoes carry the mosquito from the human being to the swamp.

In 1894, Manson applies his hypothesis about filaria to the mobile filaments. He ties two problems together. The filaments appear only in blood outside of blood vessels; they are flagellated spores that represent the first stage of the parasite's life outside the human body. What is observed *in vitro* must be what happens naturally in the body of an insect: "The mosquito having been shown to be the agent by which the filaria is removed from the human blood vessels, this, or a similar suctorial insect must be the agent which removes from the human blood vessels those forms of the malaria organism which are destined to continue the existence of this organism outside the body."[28] After the mosquito's death, the parasite must pass into the water and infect human beings, either by way of drinking water or by the old mechanism of aerial miasma. This hypothesis provides researchers with the setup for an experiment, namely to prick patients whose blood contained cells that were likely to provide flagellated bodies. It also indicates where to look, namely in the stomach of the insect, from which it is necessary to follow the parasites to their destination somewhere in the body. It suggests, finally, to repeat these observations on different mosquitoes, among which the right species has to be found. Meanwhile, the hypothesis does not exclude the possibility of revealing a life cycle different from the one Manson has thought of and a mode of infection other than the mechanisms of ingesting drinking water or aerial miasma.

One thing is certain. This hypothesis of Manson's contributes to the solution of the problem. This will quickly be taken care of by Ross. In the summer of 1897, he makes the decisive observation on two mosquitoes with spotted wings that have been obtained from larvae in captivity. These insects have been fed on two patients four and five days earlier. Ross finds "pigmented cells" in the stomach wall. The observation provides the position and appearance of the parasites in the insect's body. At the same time, W. G. MacCallum discovers the biological significance of the phenomenon. He observes *in vitro* the malaria parasite in crows and distinguishes hyaline and granular bodies. The hyaline bodies penetrate the granular ones: "We can thus consider the two forms of adult organism in the fresh blood as male and female."[29]

Manson adjusts the process described by MacCallum and Ross's observation: the "pigmented cells" are sporocysts lodged in the mosquito's body. Following Manson's advice, Ross works on avian malaria to follow the development of the pigmented cells. Their final position in the insect's body will provide the key for the mode of infection. He first lets mosquitoes bite birds infected with proteosoma as well as birds not infected by this parasite. In the bodies of the former, he finds pigmented cells; in the bodies of the latter, they are absent. Ross then procedes to undertake day-by-day dissections. Until the eighth day, the cells grow in size. Then they burst and set free thread-shaped bodies: "Then came a step in the investigation of great consequence: it was no other than the discovery of those vermicules in the venemo-salivary glands of the mosquito."[30]

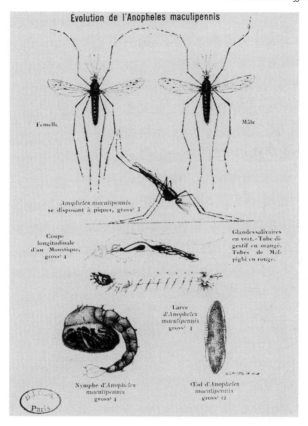

FIGURE 4-4. Evolution of *Anopheles maculipennis*. (Victor-Pierre-Edmond Deschiens, *Atlas de parasitologie* [Paris, Deschiens, 1901], plate Vi. Courtesy of Bibliothèque interuniversitaire de santé, Paris.)

Some years later, in his Nobel Prize acceptance speech, Ross would say: "Curiously enough all this time it seems to have occurred to no one that the mosquito may act in both rôles imagined by King and Manson severally— that it may both take the parasite from the patient and also inoculate it into healthy persons."[31] Ross is wrong when he says that before his own remarkable work, no one has thought that the mosquito could *extract* the parasite as well as *inoculate* it. That is Finlay's idea. But if Ross means to say that before

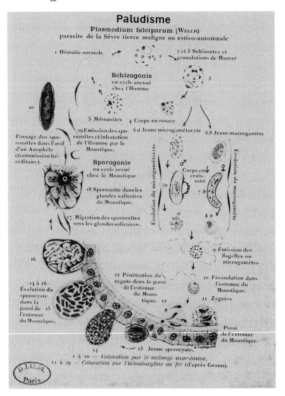

FIGURE 4-5. *Plasmodium faciparum*, the parasite that causes the severe recurrent fever of malaria. (Victor-Pierre-Edmond Deschiens, *Atlas de parasitologie* [Paris, Deschiens, 1901], plate 5. Courtesy of Bibliothèque interuniversitaire de santé, Paris.)

him, no one has thought that the mosquito could take over the role of sole *intermediary host*, he is most definitely correct.

Returning now to filariasis, we know that Thomas Bancroft is the first to raise doubts by underlining the weak points of Manson's theory. Mosquitoes live longer than Manson supposes. Manson takes the female's last meal to be her only meal. Furthermore, he neglects to feed the mosquitoes. In captivity, it is always possible to keep them alive for more than two months, provided they are fed. Bancroft suspects that the well-developed filaria larvae

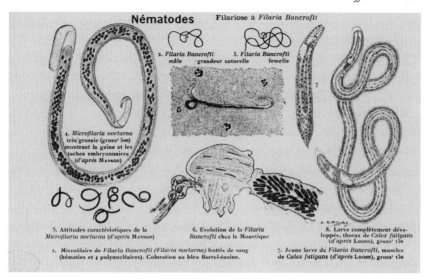

FIGURE 4-6. Filariasis due to *Filaria bancrofti*. (Victor-Pierre-Edmond Deschiens, *Atlas de parasitologie* [Paris, Deschiens, 1901], plate 30. Courtesy of Bibliothèque interuniversitaire de santé, Paris.)

observed by Manson might come from an earlier meal. Such an earlier meal might go unnoticed since Manson does not experiment with mosquitoes raised in captivity. Finally, Bancroft also shows that the embryos do not survive in water for more than three or four hours: "Water therefore cannot be the medium, as was generally supposed, by which they ultimately reach the human subject."[32]

Low is the one who establishes the threadworm's life cycle. He proceeds with the study of a series of dissections made at different times in the life of the mosquito and follows the complete development of the embryos. Essentially, he heeds Ross's criterion, that is, the time that is necessary for the transformations and the progression of living forms in the body of the mosquito. On the twentieth day, they exit the thoracic muscles, accumulate in the head and enter the anterior parts. They roll up at the base of the sucker. In their ultimate progression, they find their path: not like the malaria parasite through the salivary duct nor, as Bancroft thought, through the esophagus and the pharynx but by making their way between the lower surface of the hypopharynx and the upper surface of the larynx. That is where they await the opportunity to enter the blood of an animal at the moment of the blood meal: "The mosquito bite is the natural and, probably, the constant and only opportunity for the filaria to enter upon its next and final stage of development in the definitive host."[33] At the moment the mosquito bites, the larvae exit through the end of the sucker and penetrate through the skin. They reach the lymphatic system, arrive at the adult stage, and mate.

The analogy of the malaria parasite and *F. bancrofti* puts Ross on the track of the mosquito as vector. Conversely, a new stage of the threadworm is quickly discovered in mosquitoes and the mode of infection described. If Low is able to succeed where Manson has failed, it is because he finds in Ross's work the technical and conceptual tools that lead to an experimental demonstration. Before 1898, there is nothing that could orient research in the direction of the *Culex* mosquito as intermediary host. Manson thinks of it as the first medium and Finlay identifies it as a sort of syringe. Beginning with Ross, the concept *vector* covers at the same time the idea of a host and that of a vehicle. This new definition, which is also an achievement, is made possible by the same event. In the domain of parasitology, the description of the parasite's life cycle is equally the description of the paths and means of the disease's transmission.

The work of Manson and of Finlay nonetheless contributes to the formation of a problematic of vectors. That the transformation of tropical medicine also occurs by way of propositions later held to be scientifically wrong does not in any way modify the positive force of their research. Manson, incidentally, is well aware that Finlay, like he himself, has operated an epistemological unblocking, nothing short of opening up a new field: "Many men bring the bricks to build a house, and I do not see why the men who carry the corner stone should get all the credit."[34]

Robles Disease

It all begins with a summary description of a skin disease by John O'Neill, surgeon in the British Royal Navy. The disease resembles scabies and affects the population of the western coast of Africa. The disease is known by the name *craw-craw* and causes excoriations. O'Neill finds microfilariae in the dermis. Subsequently, Manson describes adult filariae he finds in a tumor taken from a patient—yet not for a moment does he think to make the connection with the microfilariae O'Neill had described. Prior to 1915, little is known about this new filariasis. Then, in the years 1916–17, Robles in Guatemala identifies *Onchocerca volvulus*, the parasite of an affection locally known as "coastal disease." Robles manages very quickly to relate to one another the roundworm and the set of syndromes this new clinical entity presents. But his research is not limited to the description of the syndromes of onchocerciasis. The identification of endemic zones, which leads to the identification of the vector, constitutes a model for epidemiological research. While the second part of this story thus takes the form of a detour via Central America, the third part is characterized by a return to Africa. In the 1930s, the physicians Montpellier, Hisette, and Blacklock provide proof of the pertinence of Robles's work.

African Beginnings

In 1875, O'Neill publishes the very first description of the microfilariae encountered in the skin of individuals affected by a local disease, the craw-craw. The examination of the wheals that appear at the onset of the disease turns out positive. O'Neill suggests a technique for finding the embryos. The skin is to be pinched such that the wheal is located on the fold. Then, it is enough to cut from the epidermis a small, thin piece with a scalpel: "This film, moistened with a drop of water, and magnified about 100 diameters, will very likely contain at least one filaria, easily detected in the field by its violent contortions."[1] O'Neill reports two more techniques that make it possible to see without difficulty several embryos under the microscope, namely either to scrape off the tip of the wheal, place the fragment thus obtained in water and divide it, or to dissect the wheal to detach the deeper layer of the dermis.

In 1893, Leuckart informs Manson that he has obtained from "a German medical missionary" working in West Africa two tumors about the size of pigeon eggs. These contained filariae, the females measuring about two feet in length, the males about half that length. The worms are rolled up in a ball and bathed in a liquid full of embryos. In a chapter entitled "Diseases of the Skin in Tropical Climates" included in Andrew Davidson's manual of tropical medicine, Manson soon recounts this story and briefly notes a particularity of this new roundworm *Filaria volvulxus* (as he calls it), which is that the embryo does not have a sheath: "It is probable, therefore, judging from the absence of this structure, that *F. volvulxus* is not the mature form of *F. diurna*, and it is certainly not the mature form of *F. nocturna*."[2] At this moment, the only thing that is certain is that *F. volvulus* is a new filaria since its embryos are different from the best-known filariae with which it could have been confused; to be more precise, *F. volvulus* differs from both the filaria *Loa loa* and from *F. bancrofti*. The sheathed embryos of the former parasite, responsible for Calabar swellings, are encountered in the blood during the day (hence the name *F. diurna*); the embryos, also sheathed, of the latter parasite, responsible for elephantiasis, show up in the blood at night (hence *F. nocturna*).[3]

Grove, one of the best historians of helminthology, is right to underline how strange the situation is. On the one hand, O'Neill has not described the absence of sheaths in the microfilariae he has found in the dermis of individuals afflicted by craw-craw. On the other, Manson has definitely observed this morphological particularity in the embryos of *F. volvulus*, yet he does not manage to establish the relationship that imposes itself between his observations and O'Neill's. For Grove, the incomplete description of 1875 shows that O'Neill is not aware of Wücherer's 1866 discovery of *Filaria hominis sanguinis* in urine and Lewis's 1872 discovery of that nematode in blood. Otherwise, O'Neill would not have failed to record the morphological difference that is so characteristic of his microfilaria: the absence of a sheath. Grove excuses this omission by saying that O'Neill, a navy surgeon, did not have occasion to frequent libraries. No doubt. But then how do we explain that Manson did not manage to establish the relationship between the adult filaria *O. volvulus* and the microfilaria described by O'Neill? "Leuckart and Manson were the first to recognize this characteristic absence of a sheath in *O. volvulus* microfilariae, but failed to speculate on the relationship between *O. volvulus* and the parasite described by O'Neill."[4] We must not lose track of what's essential. Not only does Manson have access to the medical literature of his day, he also is aware of O'Neill's description. This amounts to saying that for Manson, at that moment, the question of whether there is a relation between *O. volvulus* and the microfilaria described by O'Neill does not pose itself.

What appears *to us* as an obvious relation is not an obvious relation for Manson, who provides a rough and ready foundation for a project whose final shape he is far from suspecting. For those who attempted to clarify the life cycle of a number of more or less famous filariae, things aren't all that clear. Without running the risk of error, we may say that Manson's failure to relate to one another the discovery of *F. volvulus* and that of the microfilaria described by O'Neill is the result neither of negligence nor of a lack of perspicacity because this relation is *unthinkable*. Manson does not know with what pathology to associate *F. volvulus*. And above all, Manson confounds the microfilaria described by O'Neill with the microfilaria of another species he has just found, *F. perstans.*

Furthermore, it is sufficient to show that the relation between *F. volvulus* and O'Neill's microfilaria is still unthinkable at the turn of the nineteenth and twentieth centuries to understand that *a forteriori* it is unthinkable in 1893. To do so, we must begin by consulting either the first edition of 1898 or the second edition of 1900 of Manson's *Tropical Diseases.* Manson says that in 1891 he has described *F. perstans,* a new filaria that is clearly distinct from *F. nocturna* and *F. diurna.* And indeed, the embryos of *F. perstans* violate the law of periodicity and lack a sheath. Manson also recalls his 1893 description of *F. volvulus,* which, too, differs from *F. nocturna* and *F. diurna* by its lack of a sheath. The aberration is foreseeable and caused by a blunder. In the drawings that accompany O'Neill's article, Manson recognizes nothing less than *F. perstans.* The rest follows. As far as epidemiology is concerned, Manson considers the superposition of the distribution areas of craw-craw and of *F. perstans* and supposes *F. perstans* to be the etiological agent of the disease described by O'Neill. But there's more: as far as epidemiology is concerned, Manson takes into account that the distribution areas of sleeping sickness and of *F. perstans* coincide, and he supposes that this filaria could also be the etiological agent of African trypanosomiasis. The conclusion imposes itself: "What pathological rôle it [*F. perstans*] may play is still uncertain. I have conjectured . . . that it may in some way be the cause of negro lethargy and of one of the forms of African craw-craw."[5]

To return to the clinical picture of craw-craw: O'Neill gives the first description, since he has occasion to observe two cases placed at his disposition by Dr. Thomson at Addah Fort Hospital. Craw-craw is a skin disease quite common on the western coast of Africa and is linked to the presence of a parasite in the skin. The most important pathological manifestation consists in a series of lesions. The first lesions to appear after the thickening of the skin are wheals on all parts of the body. Their size ranges from the size of a pinhead to that of a small pea. Two days later, small blisters appear. These blisters discharge their content, leading to desiccation. Finally, pustules form in the epidermis that resemble small abscesses and contain a purulent liquid. These lesions are accompanied by violent itching.

It is not until the first decade of the twentieth century that physicians begin to describe filarial nodules. We may say, very schematically, that research on the pathology of the disease takes two divergent paths. For some, onchocerciasis is a disease that if it is not altogether asymptomatic, at least is not severe. The nodules are distributed all over the body, but they are found above all on the sides of the thorax and the hip region. Since the tumors are painless, Parsons believes they neither cause any pathological manifestation nor any discomfort: "As already stated, the presence of *F. volvulus* in the human subject appears to give rise to no symptoms or even inconvenience. The subjects of these tumours regard them as harmless possessions, and usually dismiss the matter with the remark that the tumour has existed for a very long time, and no longer concerns them."[6]

To others, on the contrary, *O. volvulus* seems to be a highly pathogenic parasite. Ouzilleau thinks he proves the causal role played by *O. volvulus* in the pathogenesis of elephantiasis. In the Mbomou region of central Africa, where *F. bancrofti*, *F. Loa loa* and *F. perstans* are nowhere to be found, one cannot help suspecting *F. volvulus*. The microfilariae cannot be found in blood, but they abound in lymph extracted from the nodules. They can also be found in all smears of lymph node tumors taken from individuals afflicted with elephantiasis. Ouzilleau notes that the geographical distribution of the disease corresponds to that of *O. volvulus* and that patients present fibrous tumors under their skin: "*Filaria volvulus* must be incriminated as the pathogenic agent of the local (Mboumu) elephantiasis on a par with *Filaria bancrofti* in [the case of] Arab elephantiasis [*Elephantiasis tropica*]."[7]

The presence of *F. volvulus* seems limited to the equatorial zone of the African continent. But nothing is certain. Neither the zones where it is endemic nor the nature of the intermediate host are known. The information gathered on the disease's epidemiology is even more meager than the information gathered on the clinical picture. An analogy with the mode of transmission of other tropical pathologies leads to the suspicion that a blood-sucking insect is involved. Physicians are spoilt for choice. Yet the idea to have the known shed light on the unknown rarely bears fruit. Research on the agent of the transmission of onchocerciasis bears this out: mosquitoes, flies, and bugs are all invoked—in vain.

Brumpt opines that it must be flies of the genus *Glossina* that transmit this filariasis. He relies on the frequency of this endemic among the paddlers and the natives who live near the rivers and tributaries infested by these flies. Ouzilleau refutes this hypothesis: the tribes among whom he has conducted his research live in the interior, far from flowing water. In 1911, Leiper suggests the hypothesis of a gastric path for the transmission of *Onchocerca gibsoni*, the filaria responsible for a cattle disease. The thousands of embryos produced by the female worms cannot develop in the animal that shelters them: "These young must be taken up and pass a certain period of time, perhaps about three weeks, in the body of some arthropod—crustacean or insect."[8] In 1913, Ouzilleau says more or less the same thing as Leiper: "We willingly believe in transmission via mosquitoes (*Culex pipiens* and *Myzomyia*) that abound in the region without rejecting the hypothesis of a very likely transmission via other biting flies, perhaps via crustaceans of the genus *Cyclops* or via the larvae of *Auchmeromyia luteola* known as the 'Congo floor maggot.'"[9]

Around the same time, Rodhain and van den Branden inscribe their search within the framework of experimental medicine. It is rare for the natural path of a disease to be discovered in laboratory experiments. Never has an experimental setup been less well set out. The vector could be a blood-sucking insect like the mosquito *Stegomyias fasciata* or the bed bug *Cimex rotundatus*. But this hypothesis presupposes that the microfilariae are in the blood, that is, there where they have never been encountered. Rhodain and van den Branden do not think: they experiment. First, they immerse microfilariae taken from a cyst into a bowl with blood. Then, they have starved insects absorb this mixture. In the autopsied mosquitoes and bed bugs, the embryos are not to be found. It would have been logical to conclude from this not only that the insects do not play any role in the transmission but also that the microfilariae are not in the blood. Curiously, Rodhain and van den Branden do not want to let go of their hypothesis: "It is possible that during their passage into the blood the microfilariae undergo a maturation necessary to their later evolution in the invertebrate host that transmits them."[10]

A Detour via Guatemala

In 1913 Ouzilleau writes: "The chapter of filariases is still full of unknowns. Opened well before the chapter of trypanosomiases, it is far from having been as enriched with as precise data as has this latter. In the last few years, it seems to have lost none of its complexity and confusion—quite the contrary."[11] Three years later, a physician solves the set of problems posed by onchocerciasis. Until then, all research on this disease has been undertaken in Africa. Curiously, the decisive step takes place where no one expects it—in Guatemala. In the years 1916–17, Robles identifies the parasite *O. volvulus* and describes the clinical picture of the disease as well as its epidemiology.

The first account of the discovery of the parasite responsible for onchocerciasis in Latin America appears in the newspaper *República de Guatemala* in 1916. Robles recalls how events unfolded. In the first case, a young girl presents chronic erysipelas of the face accompanied by lymphangitis. As for the cause, Robles hesitates between a mechanical obstruction of the lymphatic vessels and the action of a toxin. He also formulates the hypothesis that the *F. Loa loa* is the cause of ophthalmic problems but discards it after an examination with negative results. In the second case, a small boy presents the same symptoms as the first patient. In his case, one detail turns out to be decisive: the extirpation of a tumor sitting on the forehead leads to the discovery of a filaria that resembles *O. volvulus*. The following year, 1917, Robles gives a new version of the events in the journal *La Juventud Médica*. As far as the first case is concerned, he no longer speaks of the hypothesis of a parasitic disease linked to the presence of *F. Loa loa*, only of periodic erysipelas accompanied by fever, inflammation, and itching of the face: an unknown disease. For the second case, Robles describes the cutaneous and ophthalmic syndromes of onchocerciasis. The extirpation of the tumor is also mentioned. The third version, published in the *Bulletin de la Société de pathologie exotique* in 1919, essentially takes up the account of the preceding version, which describes the opening of the tumor: "On his forehead the boy had a tumor the size of a cherry which, according to his mother, had been there for several years. When the tumor was extirpated and opened, I found that it enclosed a fine worm, white and ball-shaped, with the characteristics of a filaria. I understood then that the lesions surely were due to the presence of this parasite."[12]

These stories are historically false or, to be more precise, they sin by omission. In fact, chance and error play a decisive role in how the filaria responsible for onchocerciasis is brought to light: Chance to the extent that the young patient shows up spontaneously for an exam; error because Robles perceives the presence of a sebaceous cyst. It is after—and only after—the extirpation of this cyst that Robles's attention is drawn to its fibrous consistency. The crucial moment thus has to be pushed back one step: The surgical act linked to the discovery does not consist in the extraction of an onchocerciatic cyst but in the incision of a fibrous tumor *after* the extirpation of a sebaceous cyst. The decisive piece of information is recorded by Aguirre Velasquez, a physician and the editor of the paper that publishes the very first account of the discovery: "After the extirpation, which Dr. Robles considered to be a matter of secondary importance, it was the fibrous consistency of the tumor he had extracted that drew his attention. He opened it with a scalpel and to his great surprise he saw, rolled up like a tiny thread, like a hair, a female filaria."[13] An operation without importance can thus lead to a discovery of the utmost significance.

In the history of medicine, patients' accounts are not of major interest. To prove the rule, it is the patient who in this exceptional case is the one best positioned to convey the unforeseeable nature of this discovery. Bringing *O. volvulus* to light is fortuitous, and chance and error serve only those who know how to profit from them. This is the case for Robles who *after the fact*, or *after a second cut*, sees an onchocerciatic nodule where before he has only perceived a sebaceous cyst. But here is Ruiz Aguilar's account:

> When the doctor first examined me, he told us that in his opinion I had a sebaceous outgrowth.
>
> A few days after the extraction, I returned to Robles' clinic on 11th Street. To my mother's great surprise, he told her that the matter was not as simple as he had thought. He showed her a small bottle filled with alcohol in which it was possible to see with the naked eye the presence of long parasite that looked like a thread used for sewing.[14]

The first difficulty Robles encounters concerns the morphological study of the filaria. The dissection of the parasite is a delicate affair: the filaria is as if stitched to the walls of the tumor. The thick, voluminous cuticle and the conspicuous transversal striation make it possible at first sight to think of a filaria of the genus *Onchocerca*. Since it lacks a head and a tail, identification is not easy. Moreover, the extraction of the whole parasite is a long and fastidious operation that requires hours of dedicated dissection work on the filaria, which has to be placed in water. To circumvent these difficulties, Robles invents a new technique, which consists in sacrificing dogs that have been made to swallow cysts. In this way, he is able to obtain, from the dogs' stomachs, complete exemplars that are then photographed.

The filaria resembles *O. volvulus*, previously described by Manson. The female is of a white color. Its body, thick in the front third, becomes thinner and thinner. A well-visible esophagus follows a small mouth. The cuticle thickens on the lips and forms a small fold. The body displays large rings that disappear towards the posterior end. In 1919, Robles alludes to the description Brumpt has just given of the American filaria. For Brumpt, this latter is larger than *O. volvulus* and differs from it in that the male's papillae

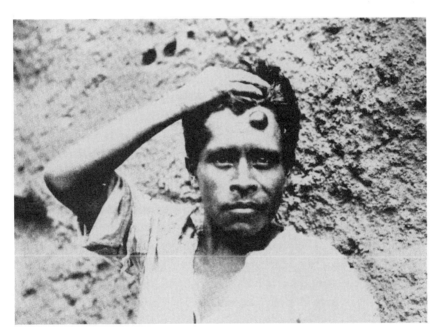

FIGURE 5-1. A tumor on the forehead. (Richard P. Strong, Jack Henry Sandground, Joseph C. Bequaert and Miguel Muños Ochoa, *Onchocerciaisis, with Special Reference to the Central American Form of the Disease* [Cambridge, Harvard University Press, 1934].)

are distributed differently. In Robles's view, these characteristics do not co-incide with those he has observed; for him, the American filaria is identical with the African filaria. The only point on which Robles agrees with Brumpt is on the size of the parasite. The female measures about 1 2/3 feet, while the length of the male is barely a foot.

It would not be wrong to say that the most salient pathological phenom-ena of a local disease have long been perceived. But these pathological mani-festations, such as they are described by Guatemalan peasants, have noth-ing to do with Robles disease. Protuberances on the head are identified as bumps: "The Indios do not know the cysts [to be] produced by the filaria and, because of the proximity of volcanoes, they say 'that volcanic rocks have fallen on their heads.'"[15] Also speaking of "erysipelas of the coast" or of "eye disease," the Indios give a good example of what we might call a popular knowledge. It consists in understanding the disease both in terms of its geographical location (on the western flank of the Andes range) and in terms of its most visible manifestation, such as the red coloration of the skin and troubled vision.

The pathological phenomena to which the peasants give these popular names are the same phenomena a Guatemalan physician called "myxe-dema." In 1908, Guerrero presents the results of his investigations in the volcano region. Following in the footsteps of a medical tradition solidly implanted in Latin America, he describes vast zones in which goiter and myxedema are endemic, zones that are clearly delineated. In fact, a horizon-tal line cuts across the mountain range at about 4000 feet altitude. Above this line, endemic goiter with its characteristic tumors is observed. Below this line, myxedemas are prevalent. Patients present entirely characteristic moon face edema. Their lips are slightly bluish. Swollen eyelids conceal the eyes: the conjunctiva is thick, the sclera gray, and the cornea opaque. For Guerrero, "the symptomatic framework of the erysipela is identical to the descriptions of pachydermic cachexia that have been given abroad by Ray-mond, Vasquez and others: our patients are so typical that they could serve as models for the myxedema iconographies published by Souques; nothing essential is lacking."[16]

Around the same time that Chagas brings to light the different forms of parasitical thyroiditis in the Brazilian state of Minas Gerais, Guerrero

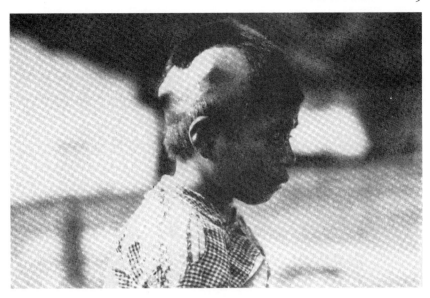

FIGURE 5-2. Illustration of the place and characteristics of tumors on the head. (Richard P. Strong, Jack Henry Sandground, Joseph C. Bequaert and Miguel Muños Ochoa, *Onchocerciaisis, with Special Reference to the Central American Form of the Disease* [Cambridge, Harvard University Press, 1934]).

reports the existence of a thyroid dystrophy on the flanks of the coastal volcanoes. Just as the parasitical thyroiditis described by Chagas must not be confused with the American trypanosomiasis identified by Romaña, it would be wrong to see Robles disease in the thyroid dystrophy described by Guerrero. This is the right context to pose a question that recurs in Latin American medical historiography. It is this: the perspective of nationalist history imposes the valorization of scientific statements that have no epistemological value. A history of continuity wins out over a history of ruptures. In this, the narratives of historians of medicine are often on the same level as a nationalist history in search of heroic exploits.

From the beginning, Robles describes the main syndromes of onchocerciasis. The cystic syndrome is characteristic. "[The nodules] are located mainly on the head, where they tend to be localized in the temporo-parietal

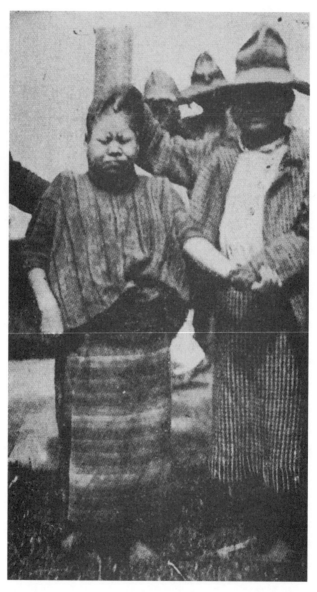

FIGURE 5-3. Acute period. Tumefaction of the face. (Rodolfo Robles, "Onchocercose humaine au Guatemala produisant la cécité et 'l'érysipèle du littoral' (Erisipela de la costa)," *Bulletin de la Société de pathologie exotique* 12, no. 7 [1919]: 449. Courtesy of Bibliothèque interuniversitaire de santé, Paris.)

region. The order of frequency is as follows: the occipital region; then the frontal [region], commonly three to four fingers from the hairline; they may be present over the mastoid region and in the skin of the forehead, but here they are rare."[17] These nodules may be found either in the dermis, where they move when pressed, or in deeper-lying areas where they can mimic veritable exostoses. It is by way of cutting into these deep-lying cysts that Robles finds tumors that are able, at times, completely to perforate the skull.

Two other series of pathological phenomena characterize the clinical framework of onchocerciasis: skin lesions and eye lesions. At the acute stage, a discolored, stretched, and swollen face mimics classic facial *erysipelas*. Fever accompanies these pathological manifestations. The lymphangitis ends with fissures in the skin that emit a serous liquid. After a few days, the fever subsists and the patient enters the chronic phase, which is characterized by a hard edema and eczematous, pigmented, and shiny skin of a greenish hue. The ears are deformed, enlarged, and bent forward. The eyelids are swollen and the lips deformed. Painful itchiness provokes scratching lesions. As for the eyes, the symptoms are very pronounced. Most often, iritis, a pathognomic sign of onchocerciasis, is observed, as is an alteration of the cornea that follows an inflammation of the eye's vascular membranes. The deeper layers of these ulcerations are described as punctiform keratitis: spots strewn across the lusterless cornea. To this picture, we need to add functional symptoms like sight impairment and photophobia, the most severe forms of which can go as far as blindness.

To Robles, the lesions seem to be provoked by the toxins set free by the onchocercotic cysts, a pathogeny that imposes itself within the framework of the treatment. And the extirpation of the tumor does indeed entail the disappearance of ophthalmic problems. Robles reports a case in which the excision of the single cyst the patient presented on the hip resulted in improved vision. As early as in the case of his little patient, the extraction of the onchocercotic tumor is immediately followed by a rapid regression of the photophobia from which he suffered. Pacheco Luna has aptly summarized the situation: "For the patients afflicted with ophthalmic problems due to onchocerciasis, the formula is as follows: progression of blindness if there is no surgical intervention, immediate recovery if the extirpation of the filarial tumors is undertaken."[18]

As far as the epidemiology of the disease is concerned, we may say that it is decisive where the little patient comes from, the region around Patulul, which lies between the Volcán de Fuego and the Volcán Atitlán and where coffee is cultivated. I will return for a moment to the patient's account. During the second visit, some days after the extraction of the cyst, Robles tells the mother he would like to visit the plantation,

> because my mother had told Robles that on the farm there were many who had the same symptoms as me, and that Indio children had their bellies rubbed with toads to heal them (a treatment I cannot remember being applied to me).
>
> During the Holy Week vacation, Dr. Robles, accompanied by Faustino Gonzales Sierra (today a doctor, too), came to the farm and proceeded to extract a large number of cysts. In the hallway outside the office, they set up an improvised operating table for these small interventions performed on all children who had cysts, who had previously been shaved.[19]

Given the large number of insects that might transmit the disease, the first thing is to delimit the infestation zone. Very quickly, Robles is able to show that the distribution are of the parasitosis corresponds to a strip of land that stretches between the Le Fuego and Atitlán volcanoes at an altitude that varies between 2,000 and 4,000 feet. This is possible because on the El Baúl plantation, there are two camps. In the first camp, situated at 2,300 feet, there are many cases. In the second, situated somewhat lower at less than 1,600 feet, there are only very few cases. Such a disparity between two places that are so close to one another can only be explained by the geographical distribution of the vector. It also shows that the type of cultivation has no influence: coffee or sugar cane plantations extend from 1,000 to 6,500 feet altitude.

To verify this hypothesis, Robles begins by eliminating the modes of transmission taken to be the most common: the transmission connected to the proximity of other people and the indirect propagation via drinking water. First, contact transmission must be excluded. The men who harvest coffee in the infested areas live in the lower camp with their wives. Yet these women have never lived on the higher campsite and are not contaminated by their husbands. Reciprocally, there are men who live on the lower campsite and who, although they are married to infected women from the higher campsite, are not afflicted. At first sight, Robles seems to discard direct contagion. In reality, when we take into account the fact that he is concerned with a parasitosis, he simply shows that the transmitting agent is not encountered in the lower camp. This agent is all the less likely to be encountered there since the smoke of hearth fires always lit in the huts made of bamboo and palm leaves would quickly have chased it away.

Robles then eliminates drinking water from the propagation of onchocerciasis. It could be believed to serve as a medium; the hypothesis of a gastric path of infection has been suggested for dracunculiasis and for *O. gibsoni* in cattle. Once scratching has produced lesions, intradermic embryos could fall into the environment and turn up in wastewater. But the embryos, like those of *F. medinensis*, could also evolve inside a crustacean to then be ingested with drinking water. Yet the river crosses zones where the parasite is endemic as well as zones a little lower that are unaffected. Even though water is drawn at different altitudes, cases of the disease are only found in the higher-lying camp while none are found in the lower-lying settlement. Robles gives the examples of the Pentaléon and Xata plantations that are situated at less than 1,600 feet and where there are no patients—and yet the inhabitants of these properties drink unfiltered water from the same river that is known to serve as a sewer for the higher-lying contaminated settlement.

Yet water can also be suspected insofar as its presence was seen as if not a sufficient, at least a necessary condition. This is Brumpt's hypothesis, according to which the presence of water is decisive for the propagation of African onchocerciasis via flies of the genus *Glossina*, especially those species whose habitat is close to rivers and watering holes such as *G. palpalis* and *G. tachinoides*. Robles opposes to this hypothesis observations that show that water plays no role whatsoever in the propagation of onchocerciasis. The infected plantations are on summits or hollows, some close to rivers, others far from water. In consequence, the presence of water, contrary to what Brumpt says on the subject of African *Onchocerca*, appears to have no influence.

What gets Robles on the track of midges are records of daily travel between homes and plantations. In fact, the workers' comings and goings yield the time of day during which the infection must take place. The peasants harvest coffee at an altitude of about 2,300 or 2,600 feet. Those who live in the lower settlement and are infected must contract the disease during the day since they leave the areas of cultivation and descend to their homes before sunset. Furthermore, the area of the upper settlement above the plantations where cases of the disease occur can be superimposed on the distribution area of *Simulia*, small flies that mimic black gnats:

> We think that the vectors are two *diptera nematocera* of the genus *Simulium*, which we believe to be the *S. samboni* and the *S. dinelli*, and which exist between 2,000 and 4,000 feet above sea level. . . . They are the only sucking insects known to us in this zone. They do not live below there although sucking insects are widespread in considerable and ever-increasing numbers in the lower (warmer) zones.[20]

Certainly, Robles simply adds an argument in favor of his hypothesis when he exposes his subjects to blackflies; yet he does not prove it for all that. He certainly does not seek to prove that the filaria larvae can be found in the insect or that it inoculates the definitive human host with them. Robles only establishes that the incriminated species is the one that bites habitually in a manner that lasts long enough for the flies to absorb a drop of blood that can be seen to fill their abdomen. After the bite, they are so heavy they can barely fly. In the most afflicted settlement, around ten in the morning, he exposes some ten sick children to the insects' bites. To avoid disturbing the gnats, the children, the upper body naked, are not to move at all: "The majority of these blackflies rested on the ears, cheeks, and neck; an occasional one over the forehead or thorax. Among these children there was one with the disease in an acute stage; his face was red and swollen. For every blackfly that rested on the other chronically ill children, the child in the acute stage was bitten by five, as if the red color attracted the insects."[21]

To conclude, Robles underscores the fact that women are less affected than children and men and names the reason. Contamination takes place by insect bites on the temples, the nape of the neck and the skull. Women are naturally better protected: their hair, which they let fall down the back, guards them against bites. Robles also names the reason why Indios are more affected than whites. Not only do they harvest the coffee where the gnats are rampant, they also are vulnerable to insect bites. Robles sees that their sartorial habits are a factor that favors contamination. The Indios are the victims of choice: they dress in a linen shirt and pants that leave the neck, arms, and legs uncovered and wear straw hats that do not suffice to protect the temples and the back of the neck.

Return to Africa

The work done by Robles and his students leaves several problems unsolved. The first concerns the classification of the parasite. Is the filaria found in Guatemala identical with *O. volvulus* or not? The second problem, complementary to the first, concerns the identity or nonidentity of the disease as it is observed in Guatemala and in Africa. The third relates to shedding light on the clinical picture of the disease, especially ophthalmic problems, skin lesions, and the pathogenic processes that cause them. The fourth problem, finally, pertains to Robles' hypothesis; proof has to be given that the incriminated agent is indeed the vector of onchocerciasis. These different problems are rather quickly solved within the framework of new research.

The first problem concerns the identity or nonidentity of the filaria observed in Guatemala with that found in Africa. Brumpt has occasion to examine a vermicular tumor taken from an Indio. He confirms it to be a filaria of the genus *Onchocerca*. But it does not resemble the exemplars he has collected in the Congo. The Guatemalan male filaria's caudal papillae are more numerous and larger and the large spicule is much thicker. Brumpt is well aware that these morphological particularities are far from convincing, which is why he attributes such importance to differential characteristics taken from biology: the localization of tumors on the scalp and the ophthalmological syndrome that evolves toward blindness. From there, Brumpt is led to identify a new species that he eloquently names *Onchocerca caecutiens* and that causes a parasitosis that leads to blindness: "In sum, the unambiguousness of the biological characteristics of the two *Onchocercae* that feed on the human allow us to differentiate the two species . . . It is certain that the studies of blinding onchocerciasis to be undertaken will show that [the naming of] this new species is well founded."[22] Where Robles brings up only the clothing habits of Guatemalan peasants, Brumpt sees pathological manifestations linked to the filaria's tropism. As of 1922, following a comparative study of the microfilariae found in Guatemala and in Africa, Macfie and Corson note that there is no difference between *O. volvulus* Leuckart, 1893, and *O. caecutiens* Brumpt, 1919. Castellani confirms this point when he travels to Guatemala: "The morphological characters of the filariæ and of the microfilariæ are apparently identical with those of *Onchocerca volvolus* (Leuckart) in West Africa."[23]

The second problem relates to the origin of the parasitosis. Is there a single center of the epidemic in Africa? Or is it necessary to conceive of an American center? In general, arguments drawn from historical epidemiology are rather fragile. On the one hand, proponents of the thesis that the disease originates in Africa point to the trade in black slaves. For them, the parasite's adaptation to its new environment explains the slight modifications in its morphology. These latter, however, should not entail a change in denomination. On the other hand, champions of the thesis that the disease originates in America emphasize the specificity of the onchocerciasis Robles had described. Following Brumpt's work, they underline the predominance of cranial nodules that cause the perforations of the skull that can be seen at the autopsy. It is thus believed that the question will be quickly settled when identical lesions are found on skulls from tombs in pre-Columbian cemeteries. But this runs the risk of taking for pathological lesions what are the marks of trepanations practiced by the Indios even then. Yet this game of retrospective diagnoses, founded on readings of the chroniclers of the New World, is an uncertain one.

The discussion of the identity of onchocerciasis as it is observed in Africa and in Guatemala is nonetheless not unproductive. It leads physicians to focus on the lesions. Hence the third problem, which relates to the parasitosis's pathognomic signs: in Africa, the parasite seems to cause rather common skin lesions; in Guatemala, more severe lesions such as the erysipela, which consists in papular eruptions on the head, are observed. Thus the convoluted question of the skin syndrome is posed. The discussion of the diseases' identity yields a secondary benefit for parasitology: attention now focuses on the skin to discover the migration of embryos in the dermis. As of 1929, Montpellier and Lacroix, starting with a series of biopsies, note the existence of microfilariae without sheaths in the skin of their African patients. For the first time, a relation is established between embryos found in the dermis and the adult filaria found in the cysts.

This discovery of microfilaria in connective tissue makes it possible to throw new light on the disease's pathogenesis. It also restored O'Neill's pioneering work to contemporary relevance. In fact, Montpellier and Lacroix demonstrate the constant presence of microfilariae in subjects who present a skin disease very similar to *craw-craw*: "The search for filarial embryos in other subjects who were natives of the same regions but unaffected by this dermatosis has remained negative. With which facts already known does this syndrome accord? One immediately thinks of the descriptions O'Neill gave in 1875 under the name craw-craw."[24]

Does O'Neill's description of craw-craw, of this disease that so resembles scabies, correspond to the pathological manifestations of onchocerciasis? Montpellier and Lacroix answer this question with yes. Concerned with clarification, they suggest to substitute the confusing name *craw-craw* with *filarial itch* [*gale filarienne*, lit. "filarial scabies"]. For them, dermal parasitism is no doubt the cause of the skin syndrome. The eruptive lesions seem to be the direct consequence of the trauma of lesions caused by scratching. This amounts to saying that the microfilariae stimulate an inflammation that in turn exacerbates the pathological condition. What, then, would be the advantage of adopting the name *filarial itch*? "This designation would have the double advantage of bringing to the fore the most salient things about this affection: the pruritic syndrome that recalls scabies and its filarial etiology."[25] The name *craw-craw* must thus be reserved for a pathological condition distinct from this filariasis, and it would continue to have the popular meaning it has in the tropical regions, where it stands for any dermatitis whatsoever that is caused by microbial infection.

On this point, Brumpt agrees with Montpellier and Lacroix: the term *craw-craw* applies to dermatoses widespread in regions where onchocerciasis does not exist. But Brumpt opposes his colleagues when he underscores that craw-craw is not neatly distinct from filarial itch. For him, this filarial itch is to be observed in cases where tumors are visible and microfilariae easily identifiable in the skin. Yet these observations confront him with dermatoses without apparent tumors. Montpellier and Lacroix underline that

Brumpt's objection is unfounded: it is well known that the smallness of the nodules often renders them invisible and that their localization does not make it easy to encounter them, for the cysts may be where they are difficult to see (iliac spine and crest, ribcage, scalp). In short, the lesions that resemble filarial itch can be present without there being any onchocerciatic cysts to be found.

Differing from Brumpt, Ouzilleau confirms Montpellier and Lacroix's observations: "The subjects infested with *O. volvulus always present a general infestation of the dermis with microfilariae* volvulus, as has been well perceived and affirmed by Montpellier and Lacroix."[26] He is reticent as to the designation *filarial itch* because the skin syndrome is not reducible to this single pathological phenomenon. There is more than a simple inflammatory reaction after a scratching lesion. The microfilariae produce a series of lesions that are perfectly identifiable, even pathognomic: dry, thick, lichenified cutaneous zones reminiscent of "lizard skin." Depigmented zones are also observed.

> Contrary to Montpellier and Lacroix, we tend to admit that the cutaneous lesions observed in vulvolosis do not arise from the itching; the microfilaria *volvulus* creates clear inflammatory reactions in the dermis that we have analyzed and that are manifest in pseudo-ichthyosis (in two thirds of all cases), in elephantiasis of the genital organs and of other parts of the integumentary system, in cutaneous achromaticity and atrophy.[27]

Some fifteen years after the descriptions provided by Robles and his students, Hisette confirms the value of the ophthalmic syndrome. In 1931, to be precise, he publishes a note on the ophthalmic affection of filarial origin in certain regions of the Congo. He describes ocular lesions that have been seen in Guatemala and realizes they are the consequence of cranial nodules: "The ophthalmic symptoms offer a more or less congruent symptomatology. In [the case of] this onchocerciasis with predominant ophthalmic manifestations, I have experienced that the ablation of the filarial cysts produces a favorable effect on the ophthalmic apparatus."[28] In the Sankuru region, situated between the Katanga and the western provinces of the Belgian Congo, Hisette observes ophthalmic problems in half of the patients that carry *O. volvulus* tumors.

The fourth and last problem concerns the nature of this parasitosis's vector. In 1924 Blanchard and Laigret are still occupied with experiments to verify the existence in certain insects of an elective tropism. This tropism could explain the migration of microfilariae toward the buccal apparatus of bloodsucking insects: ticks, bugs, mosquitoes, leeches, Congo floor maggots. All bloodsucking parasites turn out to be capable of ingesting, in the course of a blood meal, the embryos lodged in the skin. A vague tropism seems to have been demonstrated, but not having followed even the smallest evolution of the embryos in the insect, Blanchard and Laigret are not able to find the microfilariae's intermediate host. Under these conditions, their conclusion is not surprising: "These facts are far from providing a definitive solution to the problem of the transmission of *Onchocerca volvulus*."[29]

Around the same time, Blacklock begins his research on the propagating agent of *O. volvulus* in Sierra Leone. Because the microfilariae are found in the skin and not in the blood, Blacklock is led to the formulation of an ingenious hypothesis. He supposes that the agent that extracts the larvae must be an arthropod capable of producing a lesion on the skin. In its effort to draw blood, the insect could dislodge the larvae at the moment it cuts into the connective tissue. The species *Simulium damnosum* seems to be the right one: "Although this species attacked the skin readily[,] it was slow in reaching the blood and appeared to have difficulty in getting through the skin; this delay led to the belief that, in biting, this insect inflicted considerable damage on the skin."[30] This hypothesis is confirmed by an examination of several hundred specimens captured in a region where the affection is rampant. Blacklock finds larvae in the stomach and the gut. He then observes their development in the fly's thorax and its head. Furthermore, experimental inoculations of monkeys turn out positive. In 1919 Robles writes: "I believe I can hypothesize that these [flies] are the intermediate hosts. At any rate, it is necessary to demonstrate this, and it has not been done."[31] A few years later, the deed is done. The embryos are extracted from the dermis by the fly, and they are inoculated at the moment of the bite: the larvae escape through the membranous part of the lip and penetrate through the skin.

Rarely is the entire set of problems posed by a new pathology solved all at once. And in the epistemological history of a disease, there are so many factors that can enter into play that it would be hazardous to evoke anything like a paradigm of tropical medicine, such as this exemplary instance: describing a new entity, finding the etiological agent, and identifying its vector (or the inverse). Two examples, among many others, suffice to ruin this simplistic schema. In the 1880s, elephantiasis, its pathogenic agent, and the mosquito are known. But some twenty years lapse before Low sheds light on the life cycle of the parasite and on its mode of propagation. In the 1910s Chagas identifies the parasite and the vector of the disease he calls "parasitic thyroiditis." But it takes some twenty years until Romaña describes the clinical picture and the epidemiology of the disease. Robles is one of the rare physicians to have resolved the entire set of problems posed by onchocerciasis. A long time after his momentous work, Richard P. Strong, Professor of Tropical Medicine at Harvard Medical School, leads a great expedition to Guatemala. In 1934 he publishes *Onchocerciasis with Special Reference to the Central American Form of the Disease*. Obviously, Strong has stepped into Robles's shoes—with so much ease that one searches in vain for even the least reference to the Guatemalan physician.

Chagas's Error

The study of the history of Chagas disease has undergone a revival in recent years. Questions about how that history ought to be investigated have
aroused passionate debate in Brazil, England, and Germany. We witness the
enfranchisement of American trypanosomiasis from the limitations of the
social history of medicine. The resistance my 1999 book *Chagas Disease*[1]
encountered and the violent attacks of which it was the subject may be considered proof of this new curiosity about the history of science. Yet it would
be wrong to underestimate the strength of recent studies, which undeniably
are signs of the perspicacity of the criticism that has come my way. Advocates of the social history of medicine unanimously underline my methodological errors, my anachronisms, and other weak points. They have also
managed to bring to light the true goal of my research: to devalue the work
of Chagas, this great figure of Brazilian medicine. And that, in the eyes of
those who in all modesty present themselves as guarantors of "a good story"

(as Coutinho and Dias put it),[2] is an unforgivable affront. Although these historians' criticisms remain desperately mired in their own contradictions, they are presented with enough clarity for us to discern the questions they seek to bring up for discussion.

The Recursive Method

I begin at the end of the history in question, in the years 1930–35. Oddly enough, the only evidence for the existence of Chagas disease was the presence of the parasite. Yet its clinical manifestations remained obscure, so that it was possible to believe that the disease did not exist and that the parasite was harmless. Romaña's flash of theoretical insight involved a dramatic shift in the location of the singularity. The previous understanding was that parasitic thyroiditis, manifesting itself as hypothyroidism, was an endocrine disease, atypical only with respect to its causal agent. Romaña focused his analysis elsewhere: for him, the entity forged by Chagas was a parasitic and not an endocrine disease, but atypical among parasitic diseases. Thus he dealt with the nosological singularity by describing a symptomatology corresponding to a parasitosis. By 1932, when Romaña had turned up his first acute case, he faced a dilemma where Chagas, in his description of *parasitic thyroiditis*, had seen only compatibility: Chagas disease was *either* an endocrine malady *or* a parasitosis. The absence of any sign of hypothyroidism would establish that the pathological manifestations were indeed those of a parasitosis. This incompatibility presupposes the existence of the framework that made the emergence of this morbid entity possible: namely, the set of conditions allowing for the identification of a focus of the disease. It was because Romaña ensured that all those conditions were satisfied that he was able to describe the pure form of Chagas disease.

Indeed, Romaña had chosen his region well. There he found infected insects, reservoirs of trypanosomes, and infected domestic animals. The risk of confusion from concurrent afflictions such as malaria and endocrine diseases (such as goiter or cretinism) was eliminated. In short, this was a carefully selected natural environment, because it excluded pathologies that could mask or complicate the new parasitosis. But that's not all: a

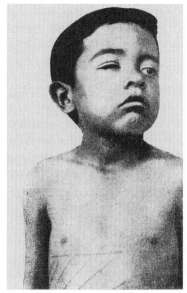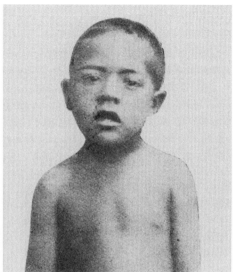

FIGURE 6-1. (*Left*). Large edema of the right eye. (Cecilio Romaña, "Acerca de un síntoma inicial de valor para el diagnóstico de forma aguda de la enfermedad de Chagas," *Misión de Estudios de Patología Regional Argentina*, no. 22 [Buenos Aires: Imprenta de la Universidad, 1935], 24–25). (*Right*) Disappearance of the edema of the eye one month after the first observation. (Ibid.)

hospital setting complemented this natural environment—a strategic and institutional advantage, since patients were quite naturally eager to consult the doctors at the Villa Guillermina hospital. Following the invasion of the parasite, pathological events unfolded in sequence. Then, in keeping with the clinical manifestations of trypanosomiases, the "swollen facies" was perceived as the expression of an edema. This sign, discovered by Romaña, strikes us as so obvious that we find it difficult to believe that no one before him noticed it. In fact, Romaña's task was not to discover a sign but to establish the framework that made its recognition possible. This revelation of a symptomatological detail, in the great tradition of clinical medicine, proved decisive: there for the eye to behold was the *unilateral palpebral edema*.

In order to discover the oculo-palpebral syndrome, Romaña needed to bring together a geographical region, a country hospital, a developmental cycle (the posterior station), and an edema, which was the symptom common to trypanosomiases already known. The result was a new etio-pathogenic schema: at the point of contact with the conjunctiva, the parasite triggers the characteristic syndrome. Then, and only then, did the concept of American trypanosomiasis as we know it emerge. In order to discover the pure form of Chagas disease, Romaña had to avoid the trap of the *Same* and the *Other* into which all his contemporaries had fallen. A swelling could be mucous, as was the case with the myxedema associated with endocrine pathologies. But it could also be associated with the inflammation occurring at the parasite's point of entry: a simple edema. With the revelation of Romaña's sign, new cases could be identified, and the disease could be seen to be a continental scourge.

Nancy Stepan, an excellent historian of tropical medicine, sees the full significance of this history as I have recounted it, but she does not see the point of my methodology: "François Delaporte, . . . in his book *La Maladie de Chagas*, argues very forcefully that the reconceptualization of Chagas's disease as a nonendocrinal disease, and the recognition in the 1930s that it was indeed widely distributed in the Americas, were results of the acceptance of the sign as diagnostic. Romaña therefore ought to be recognized as the true discoverer of the Chagas's disease. But this is ahistorical; it pushes conceptual history too far."[3] I find this statement paradoxical: my account, which describes the epistemological break effected by Romaña, is said to be *ahistorical* because it pushes *conceptual history* too far. The only way to understand this statement is that conceptual events have no history. The sticking point is quite clear: the history of the formation of concepts poses a challenge to the central dogma of the traditional historiography, namely, that Chagas was the "true discoverer" of American trypanosomiasis. What is useful about this logic is that it reveals the impossibility of its premise. Since "American trypanosomiasis" is supposed to be a *synonym* for "parasitic thyroiditis," Chagas cannot be the discoverer of a *pure and simple parasitic disease*. In other words, Chagas invented a nosological chimera, not a parasitosis.

Clearly all this remains obscure to our historians. Evidence of this can be seen in this ultimate epistemological claim: "The fact that, during Chagas' lifetime, some statements around which this agreement was reached had been the object of doubts and controversy does not imply that the research conducted during this phase (including the formulations that would later be recognized as erroneous) was not part of this process of negotiation and construction of what would come to be generally accepted."[4] Once again, this assertion by Kropf et al. must be stood on its head. Not only do Chagas's errors have no place in Romaña's research; parasitic thyroiditis does not figure in any process of negotiation or construction of what would ultimately be accepted. We must not lose sight of the fact that what is ultimately accepted is American trypanosomiasis as parasitosis. Parasitic thyroiditis, for its part, was subject to a process of dismissal, abandonment, and rejection by demonstration and refutation without concertation.

In fact, the transition from *parasitic thyroiditis* to *American trypanosomiasis defined as parasitosis* was achieved not by consensual agreement but rather by a complete reorganization of the field of research. The false cannot be a moment of the true. There is no negotiation or discussion. When we look at the case historically, we see that the false could be mistaken for the true. It was able to serve as the truth of a moment of judgment implicit in the history of the determination of what aspects of experience must be counted as real. For example, in the second decade of the twentieth century, the concept of parasitic thyroiditis, which defines a collective pathological phenomenon, was entirely acceptable. This was because it was identified as a variant of the theory of the infectious etiology of goiter, a matter of broad interest at that time.

By "ahistorical" Stepan may have meant that the history of truth as such is oxymoronic. If so, she is right a hundred times over: truth is immediately retroactive and *atemporal*. Should one then not add that truth is constituted not by histories of truth but by evolving scientific practice, that is, by the experience of science? In taking this as my subject, I was led to push historical analysis as far as possible. This led me to question a number of unsubstantiated ideas that had been accepted by most historians of Chagas disease before me. Take just one example. Among the causes of the uncertainty surrounding the clinical manifestations of the disease before Romaña, we are told, was the lack of any consensus concerning a complex, multifarious, and problematic pathology, a lack that stemmed, we are told, from the association of Chagas disease with goiter. These difficulties at the clinical level "created obstacles to the recognition of the disease as important from an

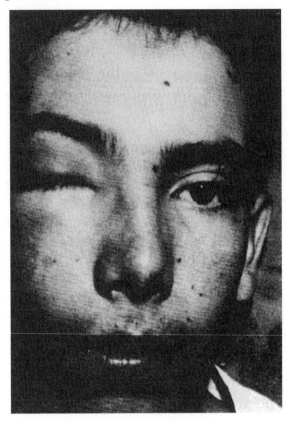

FIGURE 6-2. "Romaña's sign": The usual point of entry of Chagas disease. (Photograph by Prof. Remo Bergoglio, Faculty of Medicine, University Cordóba, Argentina [Bio-bibliography of Dr. Cecilio Romaña, p. 25], with permission from Christina Romaña.)

epidemiological perspective."[5] Historians here are victims of an illusion of hindsight: there was in fact no uncertainty but rather a pathology identified by *all the physicians* as an endocrine disease. At the time, the only question that could be raised concerned the nosology: goiter or parasitic thyroiditis? To be more precise, one should say, goiter with classical etiology or goiter with parasitic etiology? At this point in time, the idea that Chagas disease might be a parasitosis was *unthinkable*.

Such misunderstanding of my method is compounded by a number of misreadings: "It is on this basis that Delaporte, in *La Maladie de Chagas*, asserts that Chagas was not the discoverer of Chagas's disease at all. This is, however, to take current conceptions as a yardstick with which to measure the past, as well as to overlook the many discoveries and insights about Chagas's disease that are in fact attributable to Chagas."[6] To be clear, my starting point is not *current* conceptions of medical science but rather the most common conception of this parasitosis: the idea that the disease presents with unilateral palpebral edema as its characteristic clinical manifestation. Anyone who takes the trouble to glance at any textbook of tropical medicine will soon discover an eloquent photograph of this symptom of the disease's acute form. But this photo and its caption appear for the first time only in 1934–35. This event marks a turning point. The edema indicates the ocular mucus as the parasite's natural point of entry. It is the expression of an inflammation of the conjunctiva at the causal agent's point of penetration. The most salient sign is the expression not of a thyroid disorder but of a lesion where the trypanosomes contact the membrane after being deposited by the insect. What Romaña achieved was a major transformation of medical perception: an epistemological reorganization of the first magnitude.

Before Romaña, one would search in vain for the concept of parasitosis in discussions of this disease or for a photograph of unilateral palpebral edema. Before Romaña, there was nothing but Chagas's medical system. What this means is that the doctors were speaking not about this new malady called *American trypanosomiasis* but about *a different disease*, namely, parasitic thyroiditis. The definition of American trypanosomiasis as a parasitosis is thus the end point of our history. And our history is an answer to the following question: Why did it take twenty-five years after the discovery of the pathogenic parasite to nail down the associated disease? Clearly, *the most common* definition of American trypanosomiasis (as parasitosis) did not require vast medical knowledge. Clearly, this definition was within the grasp of the curious and did not arise out of the latest medical science. Precisely because the definition is common, its only value is as an *index*: it allows us to identify one of *the most novel* problems in this history, the moment when the change in medical discourse made it possible to define American trypanosomiasis as a parasitosis and perceive it as an endemic disease. Hence it is unreasonable to

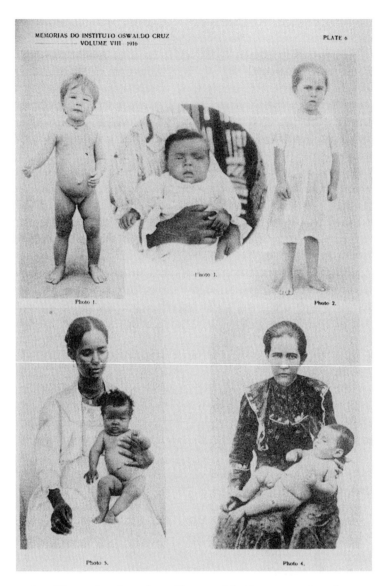

Photo 3.

Photo 1.

Photo 2.

Photo 5.

Photo 4.

FIGURE 6-3. Photos that show the puffing up of the face, expression of a myxedema: "Photo 1: Acute case of Trypanosomiasis. Severe myxedema. Photo 2: The sayme case three years after the acute infection. Attenuated myxedema. Photo 3: Acute case. Severe myxedema. Keratitis. Photo 4: Acute case. Necrotic area on the left thigh. Photo 5: Acute case. Infiltration. Pronounced myxedema." (Carlos Chagas, *American Trypanosomiasis, the Acute Form* [Rio de Janeiro: Manguinhos, 1920], plate 6. Courtesy of Bibliothèque interuniversitaire de santé, Paris.)

say that I take my criteria of judgment from current science. Furthermore, it would be pointless to judge Chagas's medical system by the criteria of current science. In 1934–35 Romaña consigned it to the obsolete past. Hence there is no need to begin with current science to describe when, why, and how Chagas's system was sidelined for good.

What is more, had I chosen to judge on the basis of criteria drawn from current science, I would have asked whether Chagas's scientific propositions are true or false. I did not do this but instead chose to describe the interplay of truth and falsehood that we see in operation at the time. It is worth pointing out that it was not I who called attention to Chagas's many errors regarding the life cycle of the parasite, clinical descriptions, anatomo-pathological analyses, and epidemiological studies. After Chagas's work became known, the life cycle of the parasite, the clinical description of the disease, and its epidemiology were all called into question. What is essential here is the web of implications that made it possible for Brumpt, Kraus, Maggio, and Rosenbush to identify what they already regarded as errors. The revision of the parasite's developmental cycle showed that it multiplied by division; Kraus revised the clinical framework of parasitic thyroiditis; and a critical study of the epidemiology was carried out in Argentina. Rather than record the absence of consensus, the key task was to show that *for contemporaries* what was at stake was not "the disease," as Kropf et al. repeatedly maintain, but rather *diseases*: *the* parasitic thyroiditis, *the* goiter, *the* cretinism, *a* parasitosis.

Thus, *to contemporaries*, it was soon apparent that the description of "parasitic thyroiditis" corresponded to that of goiter and cretinism. In the worst case, Chagas had given a description of goiter or cretinism in place of a description of the chronic forms of parasitic thyroiditis. He had confused the issue in an unfortunate way. In the best case, the description of the acute form mixed up two distinct diseases: *the* myxedematous form of cretinism, which is an endocrine disease, and *a* parasitosis, which was clinically indescribable and justified solely by its etiology. Chagas had no doubt described two superimposed diseases. The logical consequence of these errors was that Chagas disease could be seen as a rare malady or even a nonexistent one, since the causal agent seemed to be harmless. To put it in a nutshell, *Trypanosoma cruzi* found itself in the position of being an etiological agent without a disease—an "orphan" parasite.

Around 1930 the situation was as follows. In regard to the mode of transmission, proponents of transmission by inoculation clashed with adherents of transmission by contamination via the mucous membranes of the mouth. As far as clinical manifestations of the disease were concerned, all the doctors saw the swelling of the face as the sign of a thyroid disorder. Some attributed this to a parasitic thyroiditis, however, while others blamed an intrinsic endocrine disease. What Chagas had described very early on as "swollen" facies was linked by all the authorities to myxedema. And the reason why no one was able to identify different or superimposed morbid entities was quite simple: the pure form of Chagas disease could not be perceived because it was not constituted. The same blind spot was at the root of all these disagreements. What is evident *to us*, namely, a shift in meaning and conceptual level between the sign of a parasitosis (palpebral edema) and the sign of hypothyroidism (myxedema), was invisible to the medicine of the time owing to the form of analysis it used to decipher the pathogenic mechanism.

In trying to extend Stepan's criticisms, Kropf et al. merely compounded her misreadings: "It was necessary to 'wait' until 1935 for Cecilio Romaña, who, in a radical epistemological break with Chagas' system of thought, brought to light an entity that 'definitively' corresponded to American trypanosomiasis. This formulation brings out, in a nutshell, the main problem of Delaporte's interpretation. As Nancy Stepan has noted, it is marked by anachronism; based on a notion of the 'definitive' constructed *a posteriori*, Delaporte understands what came before Romaña as a period of 'latency.'"[7] I never wrote any such nonsense. I said, not that Romaña "brought to light an entity that 'definitively' corresponded to American trypanosomiasis," but rather that one had to wait until 1935 to witness the emergence of the nosological entity, *American trypanosomiasis*, corresponding to the *pathogenic parasite* discovered by Chagas. But here is the entire passage, uncut and as I intended it: "Around 1910, the identification of flagellated forms in the intestine of the hematophage implied the discovery of a pathogenic trypanosome and of the disease it caused, *parasitic thyroiditis*. But one had to wait until 1935 to witness the emergence of the entity that would ultimately correspond to it."[8] I hardly need to point out that in the last sentence the word "entity" refers to *American trypanosomiasis* and that "it" refers to the pathogenic trypanosome.

Now that an excellent Portuguese translation of *La Maladie de Chagas* is available, historians will no longer be able to ascribe to me the fruits of their inaccurate translations. Clearly, their criticisms of me lack foundation because they are really aimed at distortions stemming from their own misreadings. I should point out, too, that Stepan writes "ahistorical," which means failing to take the historical point of view into account, whereas to attribute to one period what belongs to another is to commit an "anachronism." Strictly speaking, one might argue that I committed an anachronism if one could show that the concept of American trypanosomiasis as parasitosis was formed before or after Romaña. In the meantime, it is worth noting in passing that Emmanuel Dias and Evandro Chagas were under no illusions: when they insisted on calling the unilateral palpebral edema "Romaña's sign," they were paying a well-deserved tribute to the Argentine physician's discovery.

Of course Kropf et al. are right about a number of things. It was indeed the formation of the concept of parasitic thyroiditis that stood as the major obstacle to elucidating the nature of the new disease. It was indeed owing to Romaña's removal of this epistemological obstacle that the preceding period can be described as one of latency. In writing the history of the formation of a concept, I preferred that expression to "deconstruction," "forgetting," or "disappearance." And my history is indeed written *a posteriori*. Is there a *history* that isn't? Furthermore, to write a history *a posteriori* is not to look to current science for criteria on the basis of which to judge the scientific assertions of the past. The fact that a history is written *a posteriori* does not mean that it is not the history of a "historical *a priori*," to borrow an expression of Foucault's, or, if one prefers, the history of an epistemological transformation. The "Romaña transformation" relegated Chagas's medical system to the realm of the false. Whether one deplores this or rejoices at it, what is essential remains the invention of a new intellectual framework that made it possible to see this pathology as an authentic parasitosis.

The Entanglement of Models

From the standpoint of the social history of medicine, the alternative seems to be the following. One can write a history free of all *a posteriori* epistemological discrimination, but then it will consist of little more than mere chronological description of events in a given period. Or one can write a history that proceeds by way of *a priori* historical discrimination, but then that history embeds in itself, at the beginning, what comes at the end.

One can distinguish two variants of history free of all *a posteriori* discrimination. One follows the model of accumulation. The method is to mingle scientific questions, controversies, and representations of the tropics indiscriminately. The result is a colorful description of an exciting time fraught with issues of all sorts. Stepan gives us a recent model of the genre with her *Picturing Tropical Nature* (2001). The book mingles different levels of analysis and does not distinguish between what comes under the head of scientific debate, what belongs to struggles over power, and what corresponds to different representations of pathology.

The other variant reveals that some historians are content to focus their narrative on research at the Oswaldo Cruz Institute. This is the consensus model. The term, which is borrowed from physiology, refers to the interdependence of the vital organs. In the writings of Auguste Comte it has the sense of "agreement:" of the vital and social and, ultimately, in the "social consensus" of social studies. And vice versa. The principal drawback of this model is obvious: wherever there is consensus, all problems have already been resolved, and when controversy exists, the historian can do little other than record the fact. About the debates concerning "parasitic thyroiditis," for instance, which some accepted and others questioned, the historian can only write: "We would argue that a crucial factor in this was a lack of scientific consensus about certain statements about the disease, especially relating to its profiling as a clinical entity."[9] In the final analysis, what explains the lack of consensus if not different ways of forming objects, concepts, and theories? In truth, the absence of consensus is a sign that a problem exists, not an explanatory principle.

Turning now to history that proceeds by *a priori* discrimination, we recognize the development model. The goal is to proceed from before to after. Here we encounter the positivism of those historians of science for whom Chagas is the "true discoverer" of American trypanosomiasis. History is linear, continuous, and without accidents. Since ruptures never occur, the historian can rely on Auguste Comte's resonant formula, "Order

and Progress."[10] From Lassance (1910) to Bambui (1945) progress is continuous: "From the perspective of producing knowledge, we understand the
importance of the work developed at Bambui as a milepost in the history of
Chagas's disease research . . . as a part of the process of building up the scientific knowledge begun by Chagas and his co-workers."[11] And further on:
"Although the experience at Bambui represented an advance over what had
been done before, it was only possible and important in the context of the
problems raised by the research tradition begun by Carlos Chagas. It is in
the sense of this continuity (with some differences) that it can be understood
as a milepost or watershed."[12] But isn't it somewhat contradictory to identify
a "watershed" while also describing it as signifying "continuity (with some
differences)?"

But that is not all: there is also the identification in Chagas's writings
of distinct entities where the Brazilian doctor in fact described only one:
parasitic thyroiditis. This is the little game of retrospective diagnosis. Two
examples will show clearly how to restore the basic ambiguity that I tried
to dispel. Kropf et al.: "Another difficulty arose from Chagas's hypothesis
that endemic goiter (hypertrophy of the thyroid gland whose most marked
expression is a swelling in the neck) was a clinical manifestation of American trypanosomiasis."[13] Perleth meanwhile writes: "The essential features
of the chronic forms of Chagas disease and the long-term consequences as
manifestations of what Chagas described as parasitic thyroiditis are consis-
tent with symptoms of severe hypothyroidism and cretinism due to lack of
iodine *in utero* and in early childhood."[14] From this one can only conclude
that, *for Chagas*, parasitic thyroiditis was a disease produced by *Trypanosoma cruzi* and that its clinical manifestations were not goiter and cretinism
but *goiter and cretinism as they appeared in Brazil.* Thus the label *Brazilian
trypanosomiasis.*

It would be wrong to describe Chagas's research at a given moment in
history by inscribing within it in advance what will only be discovered later.
It is historically wrong to say that Chagas believed there was a relation between the parasite and goiter or to say that he identified goiter with the
clinical signs of American trypanosomiasis. These assertions testify directly
to the blindness of our Brazilian historians who still do not see that Chagas
suggests a theory of the parasitic etiology of goiter such as he sees it in Brazil.

Curiously, the more blatant the anachronism, the less the historians are aware of it. When they speak of goiter, they are not aware that they are talking about a disease that, *for Chagas*, does not exist. Once more—and it cannot be said often enough: what exists, for Chagas, is parasitic thyroiditis.

I'll return to Stepan, who invites us to broaden our horizons: "Existing analyses miss, in my view, some of the underlying symbolic, ideological, and representational meanings of Chagas's disease in its historical context."[15] Here we have an ambitious and innovative research program. But wouldn't it have been better to begin by interpreting the meaning of certain statements correctly? This would have avoided certain unfortunate confusions. Take one example: "Chagas had noted facial edemas in many of his patients but associated them with endocrine infection and not the local point of entry of trypanosome infection."[16] Stepan's claim that Chagas noted a facial edema is a misreading; he was of course speaking of a myxedema, since he associated it with an endocrine infection. Stepan also commits an anachronism when she says that Chagas did not do what Romaña succeeded in doing twenty years later in discovering the parasite's point of entry. The only thing we can state with confidence is that Chagas associates a myxedema with an endocrine infection.

To put the point succinctly, Chagas noted something he called a "swollen facies," and to say that he observed a facial edema is to confound a concept with its referent. Stepan should have said that both Chagas and Romaña observed a "swollen facies" or "swelling of the face" in their patients. These expressions apply to the referent, which has no history. Indeed, this object (the "swollen facies") admits of several scientific definitions, which do have a history: myxedema on the one hand, edema on the other. Thus the referent is always identical to itself, but it is also different depending on how one defines it. I anticipate the objection that Chagas was talking about edema in 1909, but to say this is to forget that a word is not a concept.

Not only are these historians guilty of anachronism; they also take their criteria of judgment from current medical science. Otherwise, how could they claim that Chagas's writings contain both truth and falsehood? Stepan has this to say about falsehoods: "But Chagas's conceptualization of this illness was wrong in several respects. He was wrong, for example, in his interpretation of aspects of the evolutionary cycle of the parasite and about the mode of its transmission from the insect to humans. He was, crucially, quite wrong in some of his ideas about the chronic symptoms."[17] And Kroft et al. say the same thing when they, too, allude to the thyroidic forms of Chagas disease: "Although some elements of the initial proposed clinical description of the disease were later revised or discarded, from his early work onward Chagas noted that cardiac alterations were identified with chronic cases."[18]

But Chagas's writings contain truths as well. The Brazilian historians believe that this allows them to refute my assertion—sacrilege in their eyes—that Chagas's medical system stood as an obstacle to understanding the nature of American trypanosomiasis. "He [Delaporte] therefore belittles the importance of some of Chagas's basic statements that were later recognized as fundamental to the construction of the disease, just as Romaña's formulation would be. Here, the most important example is Chagas's propositions about the cardiac form of the disease."[19] The methodological assumptions of this criticism are fragile. To begin with, a current model, retroactively applied as touchstone, is not the best way to illuminate the past. Indeed, the problem is not so much the *a posteriori* judgment as the fact that it bears on scientific assertions detached from the medical system to which they belong. Chagas described cardiac problems, but should we allow that to blind us to the fact that those problems were also *associated* with problems of the glandular system? Does not the label *parasitic thyroiditis* indicate that the endocrine pathology predominated? It is one thing to describe cardiopathy as one of the major syndromes associated with the chronic form of *parasitic thyroiditis*. It is quite another to describe it as one of the essential clinical manifestations of the chronic form of *American trypanosomiasis*.

The criticism that I underestimate the importance of the research on Chagasic cardiopathy and the attempt to place that work on the same level as Romaña's ignores the fact that the level on which I am working involves those operations within scientific discourse that allow objects to appear, concepts to be formed, and theories to be constituted. At that level it is possible to identify decisive breaks. In different periods, different systems of thought define the conditions under which scientific discourse is possible. For historians interested in the concept of cardiopathy, however, it is clear that Romaña does not represent a radical change. The essential point is that any physician who went on talking about parasitic thyroiditis after Romaña would have seemed backward. By contrast, any physician who continued to speak of cardiopathy after Romaña would obviously be following in the footsteps of Chagas and his school. Romaña and Laranja did not make equal contributions, because their contributions were not situated at the *same level*. Unlike Laranja's, Romaña's work was not limited to the exploration of a new clinical sign. It is one thing to contribute to a refinement in cardiac pathology. It is another to eliminate an endocrine syndrome from Chagas disease. Not only did this ultimate operation entail a fundamental revision of the clinical account of the disease, the mode of transmission of the parasite, and all its epidemiology; it also marked the emergence of a new concept of American trypanosomiasis.

This brings me, finally, to what can only be called a complete neglect of the rule of pertinence. My aim was not to give the history of cardiopathy in the 1950s its due but to discuss it only insofar as it might have played a decisive role in integrating the pathology in question into the realm of parasitoses. In my history, the studies of cardiopathy in which Chagas and his disciples engaged had no epistemological significance in view of the medical system within which those studies were conducted—a medical system that combined a bankrupt protozoology with a fantastic anatamo-clinical study and a spruced-up etiological theory of endemic goiter. Kropf et al. were right to notice that focusing on the "Chagas error" led me to the conclusion that the entire conceptual structure stood as an obstacle to understanding the nature of American trypanosomiasis *as a parasitosis*. It goes without saying that a history of Chagasic cardiopathy would have no difficulty in pointing out the similarities and differences between Laranja and Chagas. Similarities, because what is involved is precisely a clinical account based on a kind of experimental medicine, or, rather, laboratory medicine. Differences, insofar as the tools available in 1950 were more sophisticated than those available in the 1920s (which won't come as a surprise to anyone). Nevertheless, the history of Chagasic cardiopathy has nothing to do with the subject of my study.

Most of the arguments the historians of medicine have used against me can be turned back against them. The task is made easier by the fact that they indulge in a kind of spontaneous epistemology. This is because they fail to understand that the pattern of knowledge that has become familiar to us since 1935 is not valid for the earlier period. It is anachronistic to look to current science for the definition of the object whose history one wants to write. Listen to Kropf et al.: "According to data supplied by the World Health Organization, Chagas' disease, or American trypanosomiasis, transmitted by a blood-sucking triatomine insect and caused by the parasite *Trypanosoma cruzi*, affects between 16 and 18 million people in Latin America."[20] What are these *current* data, based on modern epidemiology, doing in a history that claims to hew as closely as possible to "science in the making?"

What is more: our historians smuggle knowledge of a sanctioned past into pathological phenomena. Having inserted concepts into things, they tell us that all physicians had to do at the time was to recognize them there. Take the example of the concept of American trypanosomiasis. Coutinho and Dias write: "The health conditions that Chagas and his colleague Belizario Penna found were poor. Locals suffered from malnutrition, syphilis, hookworm infection, endemic goiter, and—of course—malaria and American Trypanosomiasis."[21] The phrase "of course" works the miracle of already setting American trypanosomiasis in place before it is even discovered. The more blatant the anachronism, the more likely the author is not to notice it. Some historians do not see that there can be no *natural history* of the disease before that disease has been constituted as a scientific object.

It would be useful to evoke a history of American trypanosomiasis as an emerging disease [*maladie émergente*]. This history would allow us to show how the theme of the disease's objective reality is a phantasm. We would see how this parasitosis is the result of a new configuration of the relations between different living species and their biotopes. By *emerging disease* we would have to understand the appearance of a pathology that until then did not exist, of a pathology that could not exist until a set of modifications appears in the parasite's as well as the host's ecosystems. This point of view discards the first meaning of the verb *emerge*: from *ex* (out of) and *mergere* (plunge), thus *to show* or *manifest oneself*. An emerging disease is not a disease that exists and remains unseen; that definition would have one believe the emergent disease to be moving from a dormant to a manifest state, a little like a developer rendering a latent image visible on a photograph. The meaning of the adjective *emerging* would better suit the definition of the emerging disease. The adjective is used properly, in the obsolete sense of "dependent on:" the meaning here is no longer *to come out of* [*sortir de*] but *to belong to* [*ressortir à*]. The question is thus one of a set of historical events that give birth to a disease. In the case at hand, this amounts to saying that the infectiousness of the parasite, which sums up the emerging disease, must be recaptured in terms of the singular, concrete, unforeseeable process that triggers it.

Take the example of the urban form of Chagas disease. How can an affection inexistent in a population end up settling in the city? To sum up the developments: At the outset, we have an ecological unity constituted by an ecotope composed of mammals and blood-sucking insects of the genus *Triatoma* that live in the jungle and are infected with trypanosomes. Then there is a domestic cycle that depends on socio-economic factors: deforestation, a habitat favorable to disease-transmitting insects, and water reservoirs in the vicinity of settlements—hence the emergence of the disease in rural areas. In the 1970s and 1980s, migratory movement to the cities modifies the epidemiological picture of the disease. On the one hand, a large proportion of the population is made up of migrants that have spent the first years of their lives in zones where the disease is endemic. On the other hand, blood transfusion becomes common practice in hospitals. These conditions combine such that the urban form of Chagas disease appears: the rate of positive serostatuses is higher than 20 percent in areas of high endemicity in Argentina and Brazil, 60 percent in Bolivia. This leads to a new definition of the emerging disease: American trypanosomiasis inscribes itself in the framework of pathologies transmitted by needles that define, in this case, genuine *alternators of emergence*.

We may say that an emerging disease is a disease that has never been described because it did not exist. This leads to the question of its being born [*naissance*], either from a change in ecosystems (as in the case of the rural form of Chagas disease) or because it settles in new places (as in the case of the urban form). We may also say that a new disease is a disease that has never been described because nothing was known about it. This leads to the question of its being known [*connaissance*]. Within the framework of historical epidemiology, it is absurd to speak of the disease's "objective reality." The essential question concerns the disease's forms of existence in a space and a time reconstituted *a posteriori*. Following Stepan, one might object that American trypanosomiasis was very real and that its existence predated its discovery by several centuries. No doubt. Yet we owe this knowledge to historical epidemiology, the science that makes those events intelligible that characterize the history of a given object, an object that has no history since the time of this history is also given. Yet the chronological anteriority of the emerging disease and the chronological anteriority of its natural history must not lead us to forget the logical anteriority of knowledge of the new disease. After—and only after—the formation of its concept, the disease can be perceived in a natural history. Put differently, a disease's natural history, which belongs to historical epidemiology, always comes after the constitution of the disease as a pathological entity.

Historical Constructivism

The social history of medicine uses the notion of *construction*. Few people have noticed, however, that this notion raises more problems than it solves. *Historical constructivism*, as one might call it, is not unrelated to the artistic movement of the 1920s known as *aesthetic constructivism*: a new plastic logic based on the value attached to structure. Stretching the point a bit, one might say that constructivism is useful for analyzing the structure of a painting or the internal architecture of a text. But one may doubt its suitability for studying the object of the history of science, which is the historicity of scientific discourse. Specialists in the social history of medicine are faced with a specific cultural space-time and are therefore obliged to link periods together: construction, deconstruction, and reconstruction. Of course the terminology may change, but the fundamental schema remains the same.

The period of construction is the object of an attachment—maybe we had better say fixation—that has to do with the national heritage of Brazil. The period is also called the period of "emergence" in view of the set of discoveries made by Chagas: a parasite, a vector, and a disease. Here we recognize in passing what the historians see as the paradigm of the new medicine, which leads them to value this "heroic" period without reservation. By contrast, the period of deconstruction is devalued because it was marked by the rejection of what had been constructed. It is described as a period of "discredit," "negligence," "decline," "disappearance," and "disillusion." Looming over it is a series of values linked to extra-scientific implications, which range from negative images of the disease to a somber settling of scores. It is not a period of crisis marked by the emergence of insurmountable difficulties but rather a time of dispute and neglect. Finally, the period of reconstruction seems to revive the positivity of the initial period, and it is designated by terms such as *rediscovery, restoration, revival,* and *rehabilitation*—with all the ambiguities that go along with them.

One possible objection to my argument is that things were not as simple as I present them and that it is quite easy, as Stepan says, to show that Chagas did not do everything and even that he made mistakes. This brings me to one of the main consequences of the constructivist method in history: the difficulty, not to say the impossibility, of articulating three historical periods while incorporating into the account two contradictory sets of meaning. On the one hand, social historians want to incorporate Chagas's work into a past that has not passed by making him the central figure in a historical process marked by continuity. This leads them to perceive the period of deconstruction as an episode without the slightest epistemological significance and the period of reconstruction as a genuine renaissance. On the other hand, they are well aware of Chagas's errors and have an inkling of the relevance of the critiques and debates initiated by his opponents. In the end, this leaves them facing what they do not wish to see: that with Romaña, the reconstruction takes place on a different level, on new terrain, and on new foundations. This brings us to the central issue confronting the historians: How to overcome these contradictions so as to establish the permanent significance of Chagas's work? How to recapture, in the renascence, the splendor of the past?

Stepan and her disciples have found a bold, original, and unexpected solution to this problem. The value of Chagas's work, they say, does not lie in its scientific content, since they recognize that, with the exception of Chagasic cardiopathy, not much survives. It lies rather in the discovery of *something* that cannot change, because it has the durability of a *natural thing*. The unalterable value of Chagas's work is thus supposed to lie in his revelation of the "material reality" of his object of study. The historians, who in the end concede that Chagas did not describe American trypanosomiasis as a parasitosis, think they can shift the locus of his fundamental discoveries to a different niche. What he discovered, in other words, was the ultimate referent. Stepan puts it this way: "Indeed, we can say that the history of Chagas's disease is the history of a disappearance as much as of an appearance. Since, as I have said, the disease is very real, this disappearance is apparent, historical and conceptual." And further on: "Underlying these conflicts, which spanned more than twenty years and which, as I have said, resulted in doubt being cast on the reality of Chagasian infection, were profound disagreements over the meaning of tropical disease and medicine."[22] These statements, which are as much the product of metaphysics (naïve realism) as of theology (the miracle of the apparition), assert, on the one hand, that there is presumably no history of the appearance of the disease and, on the other hand, that the history of its disappearance is merely the negation of its appearance—unless, of course, Stepan's model is the contrast between real and apparent motion in astronomy. The appearance of the disease is indeed *real*, and its disappearance is *apparent*: *something* is there, but myopia prevents it from being seen.

Unfortunately, one cannot say that "the disease is very real," because "the disease" does not exist. What is real, what has a material existence, is the referent: the *disease object*, which has no history. By contrast, the disease as *scientific object* is constituted by medical discourse. Thus one has only to historicize the conceptual events, or objects of thought, to stand Stepan's proposition on its head and say: the disease (parasitic thyroiditis) does not exist, and its disappearance was very real. Stepan therefore has no reason to be surprised by doubts as to "the reality of Chagasian infection." What is being questioned, before all *things*, is the definition of a pathology as parasitic thyroiditis. As soon as it was shown, by Kraus and his collaborators, that Chagas took *endemic goiter* to be a chronic form of parasitic thyroiditis, it was legitimate to cast doubt on the reality of the Chagasian infection.

Kropf et al. have once again followed Stepan: "Uncertainties about clinical characteristics, diagnostic methods and geographical distribution of the disease made it difficult for Chagas and his colleagues to be persuasive in bringing about full acceptance of the 'material reality' that they were trying to institute: a disease of great medical and social impact that was the object of preventive action by the health services."[23] A little further on, there is a discussion of the creation, in the 1940s and 1950s, of the conditions "for a basic agreement on the 'reality' of the disease, both in terms of its biological materiality (defined by its specificity as a clinically differentiated entity) and in terms of its social materiality (defined by its epidemiological dimension)." It is true that in some cases Chagas identified the parasite in his patients. But the idea that he was faced with *a* simple parasitosis never crossed his mind. In other words, although Chagas at times related parasitic thyroiditis to phenomena that would *later* become the referent of a *new morbid entity* (American trypanosomiasis), it does not follow from this that it was already the latter that he had in mind. Yet this is what Kropf et al. clearly intimate: Chagas, they say, was pointing at something that is supposed to be "the 'material reality' that they were trying to institute," that is, the disease as endemic parasitosis—since there would later be "basic agreement on the 'reality' of the disease . . . both in terms of its biological materiality . . . and in terms of its social materiality."

It is of course legitimate to apply the expression "material reality" to natural objects. But "disease," in its "reality" or "material reality," remains a *natural object*. And this natural object, or natural thing, taken apart from any discourse in which it figures, is not *the object of knowledge*. Knowledge of objects comes from scientific experience, which constitutes the *scientific object*. Agreement thus concerns not the "reality" of the disease or even the "biological materiality" or "social materiality," but rather *the definitions of these referents*.

To seek to reduce the history of science to the history of the referent in its pure materiality—is this not quite simply to annul history? It is always possible to project onto the disease as *natural object* the ultimate scientific definition of the disease. But, once again, this is to commit an anachronism: is it not to replace parasitic thyroiditis (Chagas's definition) with American trypanosomiasis as parasitosis (Romaña's definition)? Finally, to believe that there is something that could qualify as "the disease as scientific object," is this not to fall into frank empiricism? One assumes that nature is in itself constituted as a series of scientific objects and that one has only to open one's eyes to see them.

Our historians' accounts remain incoherent to the end. To be sure, the starting point is not an issue, since it coincides with Chagas's earliest publications. By contrast, the way in which they fix the end point is instructive. It reveals a very vague perception of the object of study. Indeed, Stepan shifts easily from the history of Chagas disease to a question of epidemiology. She proposes to end her historical account at the moment when large-scale testing revealed the existence of a continental epidemic: "Knowledge of the wide extent of Chagas's disease in the Americas really only emerged in the 1950s and '60s, largely as the result of serological tests, which measured parasitic infection."[24] Following the social studies line, Stepan wants above all to stress the importance of tools. But she forgets that it was the discovery of Romaña's sign that initially played a decisive role. Hence the order of factors must be reversed: it was not the tests that revealed an epidemic but the discovery of the sign that made it possible to instrumentalize the tests. Note, moreover, that in 1933 Emmanuel Dias carried out systematic screening in the Lassance region: his failure to recognize the extent of the epidemic is revealing of the impasse in which the clinical study of Chagas disease found itself. Before Romaña, finding a parasite by any method whatsoever did not amount to a diagnosis of American trypanosomiasis. By contrast, identifying the ocular syndrome was a way of orienting the screening.

On the question of periodization, Kropf et al. prefer to follow Chagas Filho, Coutinho, and Dias, since they all speak of the 1940s: "In our interpretation, this itinerary began with the research in Lassance, in which the basic statements of the disease were formulated, moved to Argentina, and was completed in Brazil in the 1940s, when a new generation of IOC scientists went to Bambui, in the interior of Minas Gerais. These scientists laid the scientific and social foundations for establishing the clinical specificity of American trypanosomiasis and its importance to Brazilian public health."[25] Chagas disease was an infection discovered in Minas Gerais and, forty years later, a disease clarified, completed, and sanctioned in the same place. Everything begins and ends in Minas Gerais. Once again, Brazilian historiography demonstrates its penchant for nationalist history.

This periodization unfortunately confuses the history of a disease with many quite legitimate issues that stem from a history of public health and Brazilian health institutions. Hence there is a lack of chronological rigor and a confused perception of the object of study. If the focus was biomedical research or crucial clarifications, the article should have devoted more attention to the work of the Argentines and ended in 1935. If the focus was Brazilian public health, it should have begun where it ends, in Bambui. Furthermore, it is hardly necessary to wait until the 1940s to find a clear awareness of the importance of Chagas disease in Latin America. It already existed in the period 1935–40.[26] But what was happening in Uruguay, Mexico, and Peru is of no interest to historians acting as apologists for Brazilian medical science.

Villela said that "it seems clear that the indifference to the problem of prophylactic treatment of endemic goiter in Brazil had its roots in the often mentioned confusion of goiter with Chagas' disease."[27] One could equally well say that the indifference to the problem of prophylaxis of *American trypanosomiasis* in Brazil had its roots in the same confusion. But anyone who would make such a statement would be a victim, as Villela is, of a retrospective illusion. For was it not only after parasitic thyroiditis was demolished that both goiter and American trypanosomiasis emerged as public health problems in Brazil? When social historians of medicine recognize that the whole history of Chagas disease could equally well be treated as a major chapter in the history of goiter and cretinism in Brazil, it will be because they will have ceased to confuse social studies with the history of science.

The essential point is this: Chagas's scientific discourse was part of a project whose normative purpose was to state the truth. It would be anachronistic, misguided, and careless to assert its currency. In order to reveal the full value of Chagas's medical thought in the context of the history of science, it was first necessary to take his system seriously. The test of time showed that system to be outmoded and transcended. But merely because nothing remains of it, one cannot conclude that it played no role and has no place in history. To those readers who have stayed with me to the end, I point out that 150 of the 180 pages of *La Maladie de Chagas* were devoted to the work of the Brazilian physician and the Manguinhos school. Hence there are no grounds for the allegation that the purpose of my book was to write Chagas out of the history that bears his name. Understanding what took place in the beginning was just as important as explaining why Chagas's system collapsed in the end. Why should history not be a history of ruptures? The history I wrote reveals the importance I attach to error:

> Committing errors [*Irren*], most profoundly committing errors, is the condition of life. Knowing this does not undo our errors! That is nothing bitter!
>
> We must love committing errors and take care of [*pflegen*] it; it is the womb of knowledge.[28]

1. ANIMAL BLOOD

1. Regnier de Graaf, *Tractatulus de usu syphonis in anatomia* [Short Treatise on the Use of the Syphon in Anatomy], *Opera Omnia*, new ed. (Amsterdam: Wetstenius, 1705), 528–29.

2. De Graaf, *Tractatus de clysteribus* [Treatise on Clysters], *Opera Omnia*, 503 [modified].

3. De Graaf, *Clysteribus*, 505.

4. Michael Ettmüller, *Dissertatio IV. de Chirurgiâ Infusioriâ* [Fourth Dissertation on the Surgery of Infusions], *Opera medica theorico-practica*, ed. Michael Ernst Ettmüller (Geneva: de Tournes, 1736), 4:548–71. The quote is taken from chapter 1, 552.

5. Ettmüller, chap. 3, 558.

6. Richard Lower, *A Treatise on the Heart*, 1669, trans. Kenneth J. Franklin, Classics of Medicine Library (New York: Glyphon, 1989), 173. [The English translation of the facsimile Latin text is not paginated; the page numbers given here are references to the Latin included in the English text.]

7. Lower, 174. See also Edmund King, "An Account of an Easier and Safer Way of Transfusing Blood Out of One Animal into Another, viz. by the Veins, without Opening Any Artery of Either," *Philosophical Transactions of the Royal Society* 2, no. 25 (1667): 449–51, and Thomas Coxe, "An Account of Another Experiment of Transfusion, viz. of Bleeding a Mangy into a Sound Dog," ibid., 451–52.

8. De Graaf, *Clysteribus*, 520.

9. Jean Baptiste Denis, "A Letter Concerning a new way of curing sundry diseases by Transfusion of Blood Written to Monsieur de Montmor[t]," *Philosophical Transactions of the Royal Society* 2, no. 27 (1667): 502. [This is a partial translation of a letter dated 25 June 1667, published by Jean Cusson and excerpted in the *Journal des sçavans* no. 11 (28 June 1667): 234–36; where nec-

essary, it has been amended and modified to conform to these originals quoted by Delaporte.]

10. Guillaume Lamy, "Lettre écrite à M. Moreau . . . contre les prétenduës utilités de la transfusion du sang pour la guérison des maladies, avec la réponse aux raisons et expériences de M. Denys" [Letter Written to Mr. Moreau Against the Alleged Uses of Blood Transfusion for the Healing of Diseases, with a Response to Mr. Denis's Reasons and Experiments], July 8, 1667 (Paris: Delaunay, 1667), 10.

11. Lower, 191.

12. Denis, 492.

13. Denis, 496 (emphasis in the original).

14. Lower, 190.

15. Claude Perrault, *Essais de physique ou recueil de plusieurs traits touchant les choses naturelles* [An Essay of Physics, or Collection of Several Treatises Touching on the Things of Nature] (Paris: Coignard, 1688), 4:435.

16. Perrault, 424.

17. Perrault, 425.

18. "Extrait du journal d'Angleterre contenant la manière de faire passer le sang d'un animal dans un autre" [Excerpt from the English Journal Containing the Manner of Having Blood Pass from One Animal to Another], *Journal des sçavans* no. 3 (31 January 1667): 36. [This text is an anonymous review of the French translation of Lower and King's article referenced in note 22.]

19. Denis, 497 [amended and modified].

20. Perrault, 427.

21. Christiaan Huygens, "Lettre n° 1636, Christian Huygens à Lodewijk Huygens, A Paris ce 20 avril 1668," *Œuvres complètes de Christiaan Huygens* (The Hague: Martinus Nijhoff, 1895), 6:209–10.

22. Lower, 189; see also Richard Lower and Edmund King, "An Account of the Experiment of Transfusion, Practised upon a Man in London," *Philosophical Transactions of the Royal Society* 2, no. 30 (1667): 557–59.

23. "Extract of the Sentence, given at the Chastelet, by the Lieutenant in Criminal Causes, April 17, 1668, in Paris," appendix to "Extract of a printed Letter . . . touching the Differences that have arisen about the Transfusion of Bloud," *Philosophical Transactions of the Royal Society* 3, no. 36 (1667–1668): 714.

24. Lower, 191.

25. Denis, 503 [amended and modified].

26. Robert Boyle, "The Method Observed in Transfusing the Bloud out of One Animal into Another," *Philosophical Transactions of the Royal Society* 1, no. 20 (1665–1666): 357.

27. "Transplantation," *Encyclopédie ou Dictionnaire raisonné des sciences, des arts et des métiers* (Neufchâtel: Faulche, 1765), 16:559b–560a.

28. Denis, 499.

29. Marcello Malpighi, *Discours anatomique sur la structure des viscères* [Anatomical Discourse on the Structure of the Viscera], 2nd ed. (Paris: D'Houry, 1683), 368.

30. Pierre-Jacques Brillon, "Bestialité," *Dictionnaire des Arrêts, ou jurisprudence universelle des parlements de France et autres tribunaux*, nouvelle edition [A Dictionary of Judgments, or Universal Jurisprudence of the Parliaments of France and Other Tribunals, new edition] (Paris: Carlier, 1711), 1:914–15.

31. Lamy, 13–14.

32. Pierre Dionis, *A Course of Chirurgical Operations, Demonstrated in the Royal Garden at Paris*, 1707 (London: Tonson, 1710), 400–1.

2. FABRICATING NOSES

1. Aulus Cornelius Celsus, *A Translation of the Eight Books of Aul. Corn. Celsus on Medicine*, trans. George Frederick Collier, 2nd ed. (London: Simpkin and Marshall, 1831), 11:284–86 [interpolations Delaporte].

2. Gaspare Tagliacozzi, *De Curtorum Chirurgia per insitionem*, 1597, trans. Joan H. Thomas, Classics of Medicine Library (New York: Glyphon, 1996), 1:63 and 64.

3. Tagliacozzi, 1:75, 76, and 77 [modified].

4. B. L., letter to the editor, *Gentleman's Magazine and Historical Chronicle for the year MDCCXCIV. Volume LXIV. Part the Second*, ed. Sylvanus Urban (London: John Nichols, 1794), 891–92.

5. Kurt Sprengel, *Geschichte der Chirurgie*, part 2, *Geschichte der chirurgischen Operationen* by Wilhelm Sprengel (Halle: Kümmel, 1819), chap. 15, sect. 15–16, 214–19.

6. Pierre-François Percy and Charles Nicolas Laurent, "Nez [Nose]," *Dictionnaire des sciences médicales* (Paris: Panckoucke, 1819), 36:78. Cf. Carlo Musitano, *De Vulneribus*, *Opera Omnia* (Geneva: Cramer and Perachon, 1716), vol. 2, chap. 46, pp. 336b–337a.

7. Joseph Constantine Carpue, *An Account of Two Successful Operations for Restoring a Lost Nose From the Integuments of the Forehead* [etc.] (London: Longman, Hurst, Rees, Orme and Brown, 1816), 25.

8. Carpue, 24.

9. Percy and Laurent, 78; cf. Musitano, 337a.

10. Béat Louis de Muralt, *Letters Describing the Character and Customs of the English and French Nations*, 2nd ed. (London: Thomas Edlin, 1726).

11. Percy and Laurent, 92.

12. Ibid., 97.

13. "Rhinoplastie & rhinoplastique," *Encyclopedie méthodique* (Paris: Panckoucke, 1827), 12:567b. Karine Ferret uses the term *rhinopoiesis* for the Indian and Italian methods; cf. her *La chirurgie maxillo-faciale à travers l'histoire: à propos des collections du Service de santé des armées au Val-de-Grâce* (Paris: Glyph, 2004).

14. Paolo Santoni-Rugiu and Philip J. Sykes, *A History of Plastic Surgery* (Berlin, Heidelberg, and New York: Springer, 2007), 195. The quote is from Joseph G. McCarthy, "Introduction to Plastic Surgery," *Plastic Surgery*, ed. Joseph G. McCarthy, vol. 1 (Philadelphia: Saunders, 1990).

15. Cf. Martha Teach Gnudi and Jerome Pierce Webster, *The Life and Times of Gaspare Tagliacozzi, Surgeon of Bologna, 1545–1599* (New York: Reichner, 1950), 257.

16. Gnudi and Webster speak of the year 1640 and of acclaim during Tagliacozzi's lifetime in chapter 15, "Contemporary fame and honor."

17. Raymond Passot, *Sculptor of Faces*, trans. and abr. Ellen M. Simpson (New York: Carlton, 1971), 11 [modified].

18. Quoted in Etienne Gourmelen, *Stephani Gourmeleni curiosolitæ Parisiensis medici Chirurgicae Artis, et Hippocratis, & aliorum veterum Medicorum decretis, ad rationis normam redactæ, Libri III* (Paris: Ægidium Gillium, 1580), 1:73.

19. Jan-Baptista van Helmont, "Of the Magnetick Cure of Wounds," *A Ternary of Paradoxes of the Magnetic Cure of wounds, [the] nativity of tartar in wine [and the] image of God in Man*, trans. Walter Charleton (London: J. Flesher for W. Lee, 1650), 13.

20. Pierre Dionis, *A Course of Chirurgical Operations, Demonstrated in the Royal Garden at Paris*, 1707 (London: Tonson, 1710), 321.

21. Thomas Sprat, *The History of the Royal-Society of London, For the Improving of Natural Knowledge* (London: Martin and Allestry, 1667), 331.

22. Samuel Butler, *Hudibras: The First Part, Written in the Time of the Late Wars. Corrected and Amended, with Several Additions and Annotations* (London: George Sawbridge, 1704), Canto I, 14.

23. Voltaire, "Prior (De); du poème singulier d'Hudibras, et du doyen Swift," *Dictionnaire philosophique, Œuvres complètes* (Kehl: Société littéraire typographique, 1784), 42:413–14.

24. Dionis, 321–22.

25. Henri Louis Duhamel du Monceau, "Recherches sur la réunion des plaies des arbres, sur la façon dont la greffe s'unit au sujet sur lequel on l'applique, sur la réunion des plaies des animaux, et quelques exemples de greffes appliquées sur des animaux" [Studies on the reunion of wounds of trees, on the way in which the graft unites with the subject it is applied onto, on the reunion of the wounds of animals, and some examples of grafts applied onto

animals], 1746, *Mémoires de l'Académie des sciences* (Paris: Imprimerie royale, 1751), 352–53.

26. John Hunter, *A Treatise on the Blood, Inflammation, and Gun-Shot Wounds* (London: Sherwood, Gilbert and Piper, 1828), 263.

27. John Thomson, *Lectures on Inflammation, Exhibiting a View of the General Doctrines, Pathological and Practical, of Medical Surgery* (Philadelphia: Carey, 1817), 194–95.

28. René Jacques Croissant de Garengeot, *Traité des opérations de chirurgie*, vol. 3, 2nd ed. (Paris: Cavelier, 1731), observation 6, 55–56.

29. Thomson, 185.

30. Edward Alanson, *Practical Observations on Amputation, and the After-Treatment* (London: Johnson, 1782), pt. 2, chap. 1, 46.

31. Lorenz Heister, *A General System of Surgery, in Three Parts*, 6th ed. (London: Innys and Richardson et al., 1757), vol. 1, pt. 2, sect. i, chap. 33, p. 353.

32. Claude Pouteau, "Mémoire sur les apparences de vie et de sentiment qu'on peut exciter dans un membre qui vient d'être coupé, et sur les entes animales" [Memorandum on the Appearance of Life and Sensation to be Excited in a Recently Cut-off Limb and on Animal Grafts], *Œuvres posthumes de M. Pouteau*, ed. Jean Colombier (Paris: Pierres, 1783), 2:450.

33. Pouteau, 451.

34. J.-A. Loubet, *Traité des plaies d'armes à feu* [Treatise on Gunshot Wounds] (Paris, Delaguette, 1753), 31–33.

35. Hugues Ravaton, *Chirurgie d'armée ou traité des plaies d'armes à feu et d'armes blanches* [Army Surgery or Treatise on Gunshot and Stabbing Wounds] (Paris: Didot, 1768), 562–63.

36. Claude Antoine Lombard, "Clinique des plaies récentes où la suture est utile, et de celles où elle est abusive" [A Clinic of Fresh Wounds Where Suture Is Useful and of Those Where It Is Harmful], *Opuscules de chirurgie* (Strasbourg: Levrault, 1800), 3:100.

37. Heister, vol. 1, pt. 2, chap. 73, sect. ii, p. 16.

3. THE FACE TRANSPLANT

1. In Lawrence K. Altman, "At Arizona conference, praise for French face transplant team," *New York Times*, January 19, 2006, A16, http://www.nytimes.com/2006/01/19/national/19face.html.

2. "Organs for Transplant: Courageous Legislation," trans. of "Loi dite Caillavet relative aux prélèvements d'organes" (Paris: *Journal officiel*, 23 Dec. 1976), trans. J. A. Farfor, *British Medical Journal*, no. 6059 (19 February 1977): 497.

3. French National Consultative Ethics Committee on Health and Life Sciences, "Opinion regarding medical and scientific experimentation on clinically

brain dead subjects," Opinion no. 12, November 7, 1988, http://www
.ccne-ethique.fr/docs/en/avis012.pdf.

4. Bernard Devauchelle, Press Conference "First Partial Allotransplant of
the Face," Amiens University Hospital, December 2, 2005, 7, http://www
.chu-amiens.fr/docu/dossierdepresse.pdf.

5. French National Consultative Ethics Committee on Health and Life
Sciences, "Composite tissue allotransplantation (CTA) of the face (Full or
partial facial transplant)," Opinion no. 82, February 6, 2004, http://www
.ccne-ethique.fr/docs/en/avis082.pdf.

6. [Under French law (art. 223–6 of the Penal Code), *non-assistance à per-
sonne en dange*r, failure to rescue a person in danger, is a crime punishable by
up to five years imprisonment and a fine of up to €75,000.]

7. Georges Canguilhem, "Soigner, c'est faire une experience," *Études
d'histoire et de philosophie des Sciences* (Paris: Vrin, 1968).

8. René Leriche, ed., *L'Être humain*, vol. 6 of *Encyclopédie française* (Paris:
Comité de l'Encyclopédie française, Aug. 1936), pt. 1, p. 6́ 10.

9. Claude Bernard, *The* Cahier Rouge *of Claude Bernard*, trans. Hebel H.
Hoff, Lucienne Guillemin and Roger Guillemin (Cambridge: Schenkman,
1967), 94.

10. Bernard Devauchelle, "La chirurgie est-elle encore un art?" [Is Surgery
Still an Art?], in *Éthique des pratiques en chirurgie*, ed. Christian Hervé with
Martine Gaillard and Jean-Paul Méningaud (Paris: L'Harmattan, 2003), 17.

11. Paul Valéry, *Idée Fixe*, trans. David Paul, *Collected Works*, vol. 5 (New
York: Pantheon, 1965) [modified].

12. François Ewald, "Principe de précaution," *Dictionnaire de la pensée médicale*, ed. Dominique Lecourt (Paris: PUF, 2004), 898a.

13. Devauchelle, "La chirurgie est-elle encore un art?," 21–22.

14. Sandrine Blanchard, "Victime de dissensions entre médecins, Nicolas,
6 ans, atteint d'un cancer, est finalement opéré" [A Victim of Disagreements
Among Physicians, six-year-old Cancer Patient Nicolas Finally Has Surgery],
Le Monde, December 1, 2005. "The child's surgery was delayed because of
pressure put on the surgeon. . . . Dr. Nicole Delépine, a straight shooter in the
field of pediatric oncology, . . . with the consent of the parents refers the child
to Dr. Dassonville for an opinion and asks he be admitted. After an examination, the surgeon and his team confirm the possibility of palliative surgery on
the tumor. . . . Like every difficult cancer case, the child's case is submitted at a
multi-disciplinary consultation meeting. In a letter, Dr. Dassonville recalls his
astonishment when 'an oncologist at the CAL [the Nice hospital] contacts me
to express from the very beginning his reservations about the surgical indication, suggested initially with some authority by Dr. Delépine, who is, after all,
a pediatric oncologist.'"

15. René Descartes, *The Passions of the Soul*, trans. Stephen Voss (Indianapolis: Hackett, 1988), pt. 3, art. 154, 104.

16. Girolamo Fabrizi d'Acquapendente, *Œuvres chirurgicales* (Lyon: Ravaud, 1648), 822.

17. Emmanuel Fournier, *L'Infinitif des pensées comprenant les carnets d'Ouessant* (Perreux: Éd. de l'Éclat, 2000), 234.

18. Georges-Louis Leclerc de Buffon, *Barr's Buffon: Buffon's Natural History* [. . .] *in Ten Volumes*, trans. William Smellie (London: Barr, 1792), vol. 4, chap. 4, p. 64 [modified: This English translation has "visage" for "face"].

19. Pierre-Hubert Nysten, ed., "Angle facial," *Dictionnaire de médecine, de chirurgie, de pharmacie, des sciences accessoires et de l'art vétérinaire*, 11th rev. and corr. ed., ed. Émile Littré and Charles-Philippe Robin (Paris: Baillière, 1858), 77b.

20. Emmanuel Levinas, *Totality and Infinity: An Essay on Exteriority*, trans. Alphonso Lingis, Duquesne Studies Philosophical Series 24 (Pittsburgh: Duquesne University Press, 1969), sect. III.B.2, 198.

21. Guillaume Dupuytren, *Leçons orales de clinique chirurgicale faites à l'Hôtel-Dieu de Paris* (Paris: Germer Baillière, 1832), 2:512.

22. Georges Canguilhem, "Thérapeutique, expérimentation, responsabilité" [Therapeutics, Experimentation, Responsibility], in *Études d'histoire et de philosophie des sciences* (Paris: Vrin, 1968), 386.

23. Charles Baudelaire, "The Painter of Modern Life," in *Selected Writings on Art and Literature*, trans. Patrice Édouard Charvet (London: Penguin, 1992), 402 [modified].

4. THE MANSON EFFECT

1. Patrick Manson, "Further observations on Filaria Sanguinis Hominis," *China Imperial Marine Customs, Medical Reports, for the half-year ended 30th September, 1877*, special series 2, no. 2, issue 14 (Shanghai: Statistical Department of the Inspectorate General of Customs, 1878): 9. The essential part of this article is published the following year under a different title, "On the Development of *Filaria sanguinis hominis*, and on the Mosquito considered as a Nurse," in *Journal of the Linnean Society: Zoology* 14, no. 75 (31 August 1878): 304–11.

2. "Lymph scrotum, showing filaria in sitû," *Transactions of the Pathological Society* 32 (1881): 290. This is one of the rare texts in which Manson explains the way he conducts his research.

3. Manson, "Further Observations," 11.

4. Ibid., 13.

5. Patrick Manson, "A Short Autobiography," *Journal of Tropical Medicine and Hygiene* 25, no. 12 (June 15, 1922): 159.

6. Raphaël Anatole Émile Blanchard, *Traité de zoologie médicale* (Paris: Baillière, 1890), 2:47.

7. Georges Canguilhem, *Études d'histoire et de philosophie des sciences* (Paris: Vrin, 1968), 215.

8. William Samuel Waithman Ruschenberger, ed., *Elements of Entomology . . . From the Text of Milne Edwards and Achille Comte*, vol. 6 of *First Books of Natural History* (Philadelphia: Grigg, Eliot & Co., 1849), 58 [modified and amended in accordance with the French original, Henri Milne-Edwards, *Élémens de Zoologie* (Paris: Crochard, 1834), 951]. Throughout the nineteenth century, this description can be found in most works that treat of mosquito behavior.

9. Patrick Manson, letter to T. Spencer Cobbold, June 20, 1879, *The Life and Work of Sir Patrick Manson*, ed. Philip Henry Manson-Bahr and Alfred Alcock (London: Cassell, 1927), 51–52.

10. René-Antoine Ferchault de Réaumur, *The Natural History of Ants: From an Unpublished Manuscript in the Archives of the Academy of Sciences of Paris*, trans. William Morton Wheeler (1926; repr., New York: Arno Press, 1977), 173.

11. Manson, "Lymph scrotum," 293.

12. T. Spencer Cobbold, *Parasites: A Treatise on the Entozoa of Man and Animals* (London: Churchill, 1879), 223.

13. Manson, "Further observations," 14.

14. See T. Spencer Cobbold, "On the Development of Filaria sanguinis hominis, and on the Mosquito Considered as a Nurse," *Journal of the Linnean Society, Zoology* 14 (1879): 304–11.

15. T. Spencer Cobbold, "The Life-history of Filaria bancrofti, as explained by the Discoveries of Wucherer, Lewis, Bancroft, Manson, Sonsino, myself, and others," *Journal of the Linnean Society, Zoology* 14 (1879): 366–67.

16. United States Navy Department, Bureau of Medicine and Surgery, *Report on Yellow Fever in the U.S.S. Plymouth in 1878–'9* (Washington: Government Printing Office, 1880), 35–36.

17. Ibid., 34n1.

18. Samuel Merrifield Bemiss, "Chapters from Report of Yellow Fever Commission of 1878. Nature of Yellow Fever," *New Orleans Medical and Surgical Journal* 10 (November 1882): 326.

19. Wilhelm Griesinger, *Infektionskrankheiten*, vol. 2, pt. 2 of *Handbuch der speciellen Pathologie and Therapie*, ed. Rudolf Virchow (Erlangen: Enke, 1857), §424, p. 278. On Pettenkofer's medical system, see Charles-Edward Amory Winslow, *The Conquest of Epidemic Disease: A Chapter in the History of Ideas* (Madison: University of Wisconsin Press, 1980), 311–36.

20. Carlos J. Finlay, "Is the Mosquito the Only Agent Through Which Yellow Fever is Transmitted?" (1901), in *Obras Completas*, ed. César Rodríguez

Expósito (Havana: Academia de Ciencias de Cuba/Museo Historico de las Ciencias Medicas Carlos J. Finlay, 1965–1981), 3:101–2.

21. Carlos J. Finlay, "The Mosquito hypothetically Considered as the Agent of Transmission of Yellow Fever" (1881), in *Obras Completas*, 1:268–69.

22. Leland Ossian Howard, *Mosquitoes: How They Live; How They Carry Disease; How They Are Classified; How They May Be Destroyed* (New York: McClure, Philipps & Co, 1901), 37.

23. René-Antoine Ferchault de Réaumur, *Mémoires pour servir à l'histoire des insectes* (Paris: Imprimerie royale, 1738), 4:592.

24. George Dimmock, *The Anatomy of the Mouth-Parts and of the Sucking Apparatus of Some Diptera* (Boston, MA: Williams, 1881), 15. He adds: "Now no other channel exists through which saliva could pass from the base to the tip in the mouth-parts which *Culex* inserts in the skin, and this, together with the position occupied by the salivary duct in other diptera, leads me to believe, without as yet being able to give anatomical proof of it, that the hypopharynx of *Culex* contains a duct that pours out its poisonous saliva."

25. Ibid., 22.

26. Howard, 11.

27. Ronald Ross, Henry Edward Annett, Ernest Edward Austen, et al., *Report of the Malaria Expedition of the Liverpool School of Tropical Medicine and Medical Parasitology*, supplement to *The Thompson Yates Laboratories Reports*, vol. 2 (1900), 21, emphasis added.

28. Patrick Manson, "On the Nature and Significance of the Crescentic and Flagellated Bodies in Malarial Blood," *British Medical Journal*, issue 1771 (8 December 1894): 1308a. [Repr. in *Tropical Medicine and Parasitology: Classic Investigations*, ed. Benjamin Harrison Kean, Kenneth E. Mott, and Adair J. Russell (Ithaca, NY: Cornell University Press, 1978), 1:59a.]

29. William George MacCallum, "On the Haematozoan Infections of Birds," *Journal of Experimental Medicine* 3, no. 1 (January 1898): 127. [Repr. in Kean, 1:65a.]

30. Ronald Ross, "The *Rôle* of the Mosquito in the Evolution of the Malarial Parasite," *The Lancet* 152, no. 3912 (20 August 1898): 489b. [As Kean et al. point out (p. 61b), this remark is an addition either by Patrick Manson, who read the paper at a meeting of the British Medical Association, or by the *Lancet*'s editors.]

31. Ronald Ross, *Researches on Malaria, being the Nobel Medical Prize Lecture for 1902* (Stockholm: Norstedt, 1904), 12.

32. Thomas Bancroft, "On the metamorphosis of the young form of Filaria Bancrofti, Cobb. (Filaria Sanguinis Hominis, Lewis; Filaria Nocturna, Manson) in the body of Culex Ciliaris, Linn., the house mosquito of Australia," *Journal and Proceedings of the Royal Society of New South Wales* 33 (1899): 51.

33. George C. Low, "A Recent Observation on Filaria Nocturna in Culex: Probable Mode of Infection of Man," *British Medical Journal*, no. 2059 (16 June 1900): 1457a. James comes to the same conclusion in *British Medical Journal*, no. 2070 (1 September 1900): 533a. Prompted by the work of Thomas Bancroft, James shows that the larvae migrate to the proboscis of certain Anopheles species.

34. Patrick Manson, letter to Carlos J. Finlay dated 26 August 1909, in Finlay, *Obras completas*, 6:134.

5. ROBLES DISEASE

1. John O'Neill, "On the presence of a Filaria in 'Craw-craw,'" *Lancet*, no. 2686 (20 February 1875): 265–66. [Repr. in *Tropical Medicine and Parasitology: Classic Investigations*, ed. Benjamin Harrison Kean, Kenneth E. Mott, and Adair J. Russell (Ithaca, NY: Cornell University Press, 1978), 1:445a.]

2. Patrick Manson, "Diseases of the Skin in Tropical Climates: Filaria Volvulxus," in *Hygiene and Disease of Warm Climates*, ed. Andrew Davidson (Edinburgh and London: Pentland, 1893), 963.

3. On the work of Manson, cf. chapter 4.

4. David I. Grove, *A History of Human Helminthology* (Wallingford, UK: CAB Int'l, 1990), 665.

5. Patrick Manson, *Tropical Diseases* (London: Cassel, 1898), 496. Compare p. 522: "I have suggested that, as the skin parasite in O'Neill's disease may have been an advanced form of *filaria perstans*, this parasite normally, and in pursuance of its evolution, escapes from the human body through the skin after undergoing there a certain measure of developmental advance. Further investigations on this subject are much wanted." What Manson writes in 1898 remains current in the second edition of *Tropical Diseases*, published in 1900. In the fourth edition of 1909, Manson recognizes (on p. 795) that *F. perstans* is a nonpathogenic parasite.

6. Allan C. Parsons, "*Filaria volvulus* Leuckart, Its Distribution, Structure and Pathological Effects," *Parasitology* 1, no. 4 (December 1908): 366–67. See also William Thomas Prout, "A Filaria Found in Sierra Leone? *Filaria volvulus* (Leuckart)," *British Medical Journal*, no. 2091 (26 January 1901): 209: "The clinical history of the case showed nothing remarkable."

7. François-Marie-Frédéric Ouzilleau, "Les filaires humaines de la région du M'Bomou (Afrique équatoriale française). Pathogénie de l'éléphantiasis de cette région. Rôle de la *Filaria volvulus*," *Bulletin de la Société de pathologie exotique* 6, no. 1 (1913): 88. See also A. Dubois, "Le rôle pathogène de Onchocerca volvulus Leuckart," *Bulletin de la Société de pathologie exotique* 9, no. 5 (1916): 305–9. I should specify that in 1910, Alcide Railliet and Albert Joseph

Lucien Henry transfer the worm from the genus *Filaria de Müller* to the genus *Onchocerca*, which Diesing suggested in 1841 to accommodate the animal parasite *O. reticulata*. *Onchocerca* names roundworms with a hook-shaped posterior.

8. Robert Thomson Leiper, "Onchocerciasis in cattle, with special reference to the structure and bionomic characters of the parasite," *Journal of Tropical Medicine and Hygiene* 14 (15 March 1911; repr. Amsterdam: Swets & Zeitlinger, 1965): 91b.

9. François-Marie-Frédéric Ouzilleau, "L'éléphantiasis et les filarioses dans le M'Bomou (Haut-Oubangui). Rôle de la 'Filaria Volvulus' (Suite)," *Annales d'hygiène et de médecine coloniales*, no. 16 (1913): 709.

10. J. Rodhain and F. van den Branden, "Recherches diverses sur la *Filaria (Onchocerca) volvulus*," *Bulletin de la Société de pathologie exotique* 9, no. 5 (1916): 196.

11. Ouzilleau, "L'éléphantiasis dans le M'Bomou," 688.

12. Rodolfo Robles, "Onchocercose humaine au Guatemala produisant la cécité et 'l'érysipèle du littoral' (Erisipela de la costa)," *Bulletin de la Société de pathologie exotique* 12, no. 7 (1919): 444. The first version of the article is a newspaper interview, published underneath the headline "Una enfermedad nueva en el continente ha sido diagnosticada en Guatemala" in *La Republica de Guatemala* on December 29, 1916 (repr. in Horacio Figueroa Marroquin, *Historia de la enfermedad de Robles en America y de su descubrimiento en Guatemala* [Guatemala City: Luz, 1963], 59–65). A second version, this time in the form of a summary, by Victor Manuel Calderón, of a lecture by Robles is published the following year ("Enfermedad Nueva en Guatemala," *La Juventud Médica* 17, no. 18 (August 1917); repr. in Asociación Oftalmológica de Guatemala, *Oncocercosis (Enfermedad de Robles): Homenaje al tercer congreso pan-americano de oftalmología* [Guatemala City: Universidad de San Carlos, 1947], 27–39). [The second version is translated in part as "A New Disease in Guatemala" and included in Kean, ed., *Tropical Medicine and Parasitology*, 446–51. In what follows, quotes are taken from this translation wherever this second version, as noted by Delaporte, is identical with the third version. This first quote is taken from page 447a.]

13. Robles, "Una enfermedad nueva en el continente," Figueroa Marroquin, 67.

14. Alberto Ruiz Aguilar, letter to Horacio Figueroa Marroquin dated 5 October 1961 (in Figueroa Marroquin, 73–74). Ruiz Aguilar is the patient on whom Robles discovers the worm in March 1915. Historians tend to simplify the story. To give just one example: "When Dr. Robles operated on the first onchocercoma, removing a certain small tumor from the head of a child who came from a farm infested with the disease, he suspected the parasitic nature of

this pathology since he encountered a fibrous skein inside this tumor," J. Romeo de León, "Entomología de la Oncocercosis," in *Oncocercosis (Enfermedad de Robles)*, 147.

15. Robles, "Onchocercose humaine," 445.

16. Pastor Guerrero, *El Bocio, los mixedemas y el cretinismo en las montañas guatemaltecas* (La Antigua, Tp. Internacional, 1908), 29; an excerpt from this text can be found in Figueroa Marroquin, 76–77. Immediately following the publication of Robles's work, a controversy arose between partisans of the parasitic theory and supporters of the myxedema theory. For a sample of the views advocated, see E. Quintana, "Un problema de semiotica nacional," *La Juventud Médica* 18 (1921): 214–15, 365–66; A. Reti, "Bocio, Mixedema y Filaria," *La Juventud Médica* 19 (1922): 225, 471–74; S. C. Fletes, "La Onchocerca y el Mixedema," *La Juventud Médica* 21 (1923): 230–31, 551–52.

17. Robles, "Onchocercose humaine," 454.

18. Rafael Pacheco Luna, "Appendice. Lésions oculaires d'après le Dr Pancheco [*sic*]," *Bulletin de la Société de pathologie exotique* 12, no. 7 (1919): 463. Cf. *idem*., "Apuntes preliminares sobre los trastornos de la visión observados en Guatemala en los enfermos portadores de ciertos tumores filariosos," *La Juventud Médica* 17 (1917): 241–48; "Disturbances of vision in patients harboring certain filarial tumour," *American Journal of Ophthalmology* 2, no. 11 (November 1919): 793–96; and finally, Victor Manuel Calderón, *Contribución al estudio del Filarido Onchocerca, sp. Dr Robles 1915, y de las enfermedades que produce*, doctoral thesis (Guatemala, 1920).

19. Ruiz Aguilar in Figueroa Marroquin, 74.

20. Robles, "Onchocercose humaine," 448, Kean, 449b [amended and modified].

21. Robles, "Onchocercose humaine," 448–49, Kean, 449b [modified].

22. Émile Brumpt, "Une nouvelle filaire pathogène parasite de l'homme (*Onchocerca caecutiens* n. sp.)," *Bulletin de la Société de pathologie exotique* 12, no. 7 (1919): 471–72.

23. Aldo Castellani, "Observations on Some Diseases of Central America," *Journal of Tropical Medicine and Hygiene* 28 (1925): 2b.

24. J. Montpellier and A. Lacroix, "Le Craw-Craw ou Gale filarienne; son origine dans les kystes sous-cutanés à *Onchocerca volvulus*," *Bulletin de la Société de pathologie exotique* 13, no. 4 (1920): 310. See also J. Montpellier, Deguillon, and A. Lacroix, "La gale filarienne est-elle bien une manifestation de volvulose?" *Bulletin de la Société de pathologie exotique* 13, no. 7 (1920): 530–35.

25. Montpellier and Lacroix, 310.

26. François Ouzilleau, Jean Laigret, and Gustave Cyrille Pierre Lefrou, "Contribution à l'étude de l'*Onchocerca volvulus*," *Bulletin de la Société de pathologie exotique* 14, no. 10 (1921): 725 [emphasis Delaporte]. See also Émile

Brumpt, "Au sujet des rapports entre l'*Onchocerca volvulus* et la gale filarienne," *Bulletin de la Société de pathologie exotique* 13, no. 7 (1920): 535–39.

27. Ouzilleau et al., "Contribution," 728.

28. Jean Hisette, "Sur l'existence d'affections oculaires importantes d'origine filarienne dans certains territoires du Congo," *Annales de la Société belge de médecine tropicale* 11 (1931): 45–46. The following year, he refines his observations on this major symptom of onchocerciasis; see his "Mémoire sur l'*Onchocerca volvulus* 'Leuckart' et ses manifestations oculaires au Congo belge," *Annales de la Société belge de médecine tropicale* 12 (1932): 433–529.

29. Maurice Blanchard and Jean Laigret, "Recherches sur la transmission d'*Onchocerca volvulus* par divers parasites hématophages," *Bulletin de la Société de pathologie exotique* 17, no. 5 (1924): 417.

30. Donald Breadalbane Blacklock, "The Insect Transmission of *Onchocerca volvulus* (Leuckart, 1893): The Cause of Worm Nodules in Man in Africa," *British Medical Journal*, no. 3446 (27 January 1927): 130b [repr. in Kean, 451–57, quote on p. 454b]; cf. his article "The development of *Onchocerca volvulus* in *Simulium damnosum*," *Annals of Tropical Medicine and Parasitology* 20, no. 1 (1926): 1–48. Dry reports that several Kenyan tribes have long associated river blindness with simulia bites; see F. W. Dry, "Trypanosomiasis in the Absence of Tsetses, and a Human Disease Possibility Carried by *Simulium* in Kenya Colony," *Bulletin of Entomological Research* 12 (1921): 233–38. On this point, see George S. Nelson, "Human Onchocerciasis: Notes on the History, the Parasite and the Life Cycle," *Annals of Tropical Medicine and Parasitology* 85, no. 1 (1991): 85a–b.

31. Robles, "Onchocercose humaine," 450 [Kean, 450b].

6. CHAGAS'S ERROR

This chapter was translated by Arthur Goldhammer.

1. François Delaporte, *Chagas Disease: History of a Continent's Scourge*, trans. Arthur Goldhammer (New York: Fordham University Press, 2012).

2. Marilia Coutinho and João Carlos Pinto Dias, "A Reason to Celebrate: The Saga of Brazilian Chagologists," *Ciência e Cultura: Journal of the Brazilian Association of the Advancement of Science* 51, nos. 5–6 (September–December 1999): 394.

3. Nancy Stepan, *Picturing Tropical Nature* (Ithaca, NY: Cornell University Press, 2001), 270n51.

4. Simone Petraglia Kropf, Nara Azevedo, and Luiz Otávio Ferreira, "Biomedical Research and Public Health in Brazil: The Case of Chagas' Disease (1909–50)," *Journal of the Society for the Social History of Medicine* 16, no. 1 (April 2003): 128.

5. Ibid., 119.

6. Stepan, 270n43.

7. Kropf et al., 128.

8. Delaporte, 18.

9. Kropf et al., 118.

10. [The motto figures prominently on the title pages of Comte's publications for the *Société positiviste*.]

11. Kropf et al., 127.

12. Ibid., 129

13. Ibid., 118–19.

14. Matthias Perleth, "The Discovery of Chagas' Disease and the Formation of the Early Chagas' Disease Concept," *History and Philosophy of the Life Sciences* 19 (1997): 233.

15. Stepan, 183.

16. Ibid., 270n51.

17. Ibid., 190.

18. Kropf et al., 116. The authors may object that they wrote "later" and therefore intended no judgment, but to bring an "after" to bear in order to appreciate a "before" is to make a judgment *a posteriori*. Indeed, they add this judicious comment (note 21): "Currently, the chronic phase of the disease is understood to include the indeterminate, cardiac, and digestive forms."

19. Ibid., 129.

20. Ibid., 111; cf. Stepan: "Identified in 1909 as a disease completely new to medicine by the Brasilian medical researcher Carlos Chagas—hence its popular name—Chagas's disease has been characterized as 'one of the most important infectious diseases in the New World'" (181).

21. Coutinho and Dias, 395.

22. Stepan, 182–83.

23. Kropf et al., 120.

24. Stepan, 270n51.

25. Kropf et al., 115. There is reason to doubt that the work of the physicians at Bambui was decisive in ending the controversy over the clinical manifestations of the disease. The questions were resolved by the Argentines in 1935.

26. In 1946, Emmanuel Dias published "Acerca de 254 casos da doença de Chagas comprovados em Minas Gerais" [On 254 Proven Cases of Chagas Disease in Minas Geraes], *Brasil Medico* 60: 41–43. Ten years earlier, Salvador Mazza had published "Nota a proposito de 240 casos de formas agudas de Enfermedad de Chagas comprobadas en el pais por la MEPRA *(Misión de Estudios de Patología Regional Argentina)*" [A Note Concerning 240 Cases of Acute

Forms of Chagas Disease Tested in the Country by the MEPRA (Argentine Regional Pathologies Study Mission)], *Prensa Medica Argentina*, July 21, 1937.

27. Eurico de Azevedo Villela, "Bocio endémico," *Revista brasileira de medicina* 10, no. 3 (March 1953): 211.

28. Friedrich Nietzsche, *Sämtliche Werke: Kritische Studienausgabe in 15 Bänden*, ed. Giorgio Colli and Mazzino Montinari (Munich: Deutscher Taschenbuch Verlag, 1999), 9:504, aphorism 11.[162].

forms of living

Stefanos Geroulanos and Todd Meyers, *series editors*

Georges Canguilhem, *Knowledge of Life*. Translated by Stefanos Geroulanos and Daniela Ginsburg, Introduction by Paola Marrati and Todd Meyers.

Henri Atlan, *Selected Writings: On Self-Organization, Philosophy, Bioethics, and Judaism*. Edited and with an Introduction by Stefanos Geroulanos and Todd Meyers.

Jonathan Strauss, *Human Remains: Medicine, Death, and Desire in Nineteenth-Century Paris*.

Georges Canguilhem, *Writings on Medicine*. Translated and with an Introduction by Stefanos Geroulanos and Todd Meyers.

Juan Manuel Garrido, *On Time, Being, and Hunger: Challenging the Traditional Way of Thinking Life*.

Catherine Malabou, *The New Wounded: From Neurosis to Brain Damage*. Translated by Steven Miller.

François Delaporte, *Chagas Disease: History of a Continent's Scourge*. Translated by Arthur Goldhammer.

Pamela Reynolds, *War in Worcester: Youth and the Apartheid State*.

François Delaporte, *Figures of Medicine: Blood, Face Transplants, Parasites*. Translated by Nils F. Schott.